Low Uric Acid Diet Cookbook

+ (6-Week Meal Plan)

"105 Nutrient-Rich Recipes for Low-Purine Dishes to Fight Gout, Plus Expert Tips"

Patricia D. Miller

Copyright © 2024

Patricia D. Miller

TABLE OF CONTENTS

Patricia D. Miller

INTRODUCTION

1. Understanding Uric Acid and Its Role in the Body

Introduction to Uric Acid

Uric acid is a naturally occurring substance in the human body, formed when purines—substances found in many foods and also produced by the body—are broken down. Purines are found in high amounts in certain foods like red meat, shellfish, and certain types of fish, as well as in some beverages like alcohol, especially beer. When purines are metabolized, uric acid is created as a waste product.

The Production and Elimination of Uric Acid

In a healthy individual, uric acid dissolves in the blood and travels to the kidneys, from where it is excreted in urine. Normally, the body maintains a balance by producing an amount of uric acid that corresponds to the amount it eliminates. However, when this balance is disrupted, either by producing too much uric acid or not excreting enough, uric acid can accumulate in the blood. This condition is known as hyperuricemia.

Functions of Uric Acid in the Body

Despite its potential to cause problems when in excess, uric acid has certain beneficial roles:

- **Antioxidant Properties:** Uric acid acts as an antioxidant, helping to neutralize free radicals in the body. Free radicals are unstable molecules that can damage cells, contributing to aging and diseases like cancer.
- **Brain Function:** Some research suggests that uric acid might have a role in brain function, possibly offering neuroprotective effects. Higher levels of uric acid have been associated with lower risks of neurodegenerative diseases like Parkinson's and Alzheimer's in some studies.

Hyperuricemia and Its Consequences

When uric acid levels are too high, they can lead to various health problems:

- **Gout:** This is a type of arthritis characterized by sudden, severe attacks of pain, redness, and tenderness in joints. It is caused by the deposition of urate crystals in the joints.
- **Kidney Stones:** Uric acid can form crystals in the kidneys, leading to stones that can cause severe pain and urinary issues.
- **Chronic Kidney Disease:** Persistent high levels of uric acid can lead to kidney damage over time.
- **Cardiovascular Diseases:** Hyperuricemia has been linked to increased risks of hypertension, heart disease, and stroke.

Regulating Uric Acid Levels

Maintaining balanced uric acid levels is crucial for health. This can be achieved through dietary management, hydration, and sometimes medication. A low uric acid diet focuses on reducing the intake of high-purine foods and beverages while emphasizing hydration and foods that help in the excretion of uric acid.

2. The Health Implications of High Uric Acid Levels

Introduction to Hyperuricemia

Hyperuricemia refers to the condition where there is an excess of uric acid in the blood. While uric acid itself is a normal metabolic product, its excessive accumulation can lead to a host of health issues. Understanding the implications of high uric acid levels is critical for preventing and managing associated conditions.

Gout and Its Impact

Gout is one of the most well-known conditions associated with high uric acid levels. It is characterized by:

- **Severe Joint Pain:** Gout attacks are sudden and often occur at night. The pain is intense and can make even the weight of a bedsheet unbearable.
- **Inflammation and Redness:** The affected joints become swollen, red, and warm.

- **Recurring Attacks:** Without management, gout can become a chronic condition, leading to frequent attacks and potentially tophi formation—hard uric acid deposits under the skin.

Kidney Stones and Renal Health

High uric acid levels can lead to the formation of kidney stones. These stones can cause:

- **Severe Pain:** Stones can block parts of the urinary tract, causing excruciating pain that radiates to the back and lower abdomen.
- **Urinary Issues:** Difficulty in urination, frequent urges, and even blood in the urine can occur.
- **Kidney Damage:** Over time, recurring stones can cause damage to the kidneys, leading to chronic kidney disease.

Cardiovascular Risks

Emerging research links hyperuricemia to cardiovascular issues:

- **Hypertension:** High uric acid levels are associated with an increased risk of high blood pressure, which is a major risk factor for heart disease.
- **Heart Disease and Stroke:** There is a correlation between elevated uric acid levels and an increased risk of heart attacks and strokes. This might be due to the inflammatory and oxidative stress associated with high uric acid.

Metabolic Syndrome and Diabetes

High uric acid levels are often found in individuals with metabolic syndrome, which includes:

- **Obesity:** Particularly abdominal obesity.
- **Insulin Resistance:** Leading to type 2 diabetes.
- **Dyslipidemia:** Unhealthy cholesterol and triglyceride levels.
- **Hypertension:** As mentioned earlier.

Other Potential Health Issues

Beyond the primary conditions, high uric acid levels can contribute to:

- **Osteoarthritis:** Some studies suggest a link between uric acid and joint degeneration.
- **Mental Health:** Chronic pain and inflammation from conditions like gout can impact mental well-being, leading to stress, anxiety, and depression.

Managing High Uric Acid Levels

Addressing hyperuricemia involves:

- **Dietary Changes:** Reducing purine-rich foods, increasing hydration, and incorporating foods that help reduce uric acid levels.
- **Medications:** In some cases, medications like allopurinol or febuxostat are prescribed to help lower uric acid levels.
- **Lifestyle Modifications:** Weight management, regular exercise, and avoiding alcohol can all help in managing uric acid levels effectively.

3. The Science Behind a Low Uric Acid Diet

Introduction to Dietary Management

A low uric acid diet is designed to help manage and prevent conditions related to hyperuricemia. The science behind this diet revolves around understanding purines, how they are metabolized into uric acid, and how dietary choices can influence uric acid levels.

Purines and Their Metabolism

Purines are naturally occurring substances found in many foods and also produced by the body. When purines are broken down, uric acid is formed as a byproduct. Therefore, a key strategy in managing uric acid levels is to reduce the intake of high-purine foods.

High-Purine Foods

Certain foods are particularly high in purines, such as:

- **Red Meat:** Beef, lamb, and pork are known for their high purine content.
- **Organ Meats:** Liver, kidney, and other organ meats are very rich in purines.

- **Seafood:** Shellfish, sardines, and anchovies are high-purine seafood options.
- **Certain Vegetables:** Asparagus, spinach, and mushrooms have higher purine levels compared to other vegetables.
- **Alcohol:** Especially beer, which contains yeast, a high-purine component.

Foods That Help Reduce Uric Acid

On the flip side, some foods can help manage and reduce uric acid levels:

- **Low-Purine Vegetables:** Most vegetables are low in purines and can be consumed freely.
- **Dairy Products:** Low-fat dairy has been shown to help lower uric acid levels.
- **Fruits:** Cherries, in particular, have been found to lower uric acid and reduce gout attacks.
- **Whole Grains:** Foods like oats, brown rice, and barley are low in purines and beneficial for overall health.
- **Hydration:** Drinking plenty of water helps the kidneys flush out uric acid more effectively.

Mechanisms of Uric Acid Reduction

The mechanisms through which diet influences uric acid levels include:

i. **Reduced Purine Intake:** Directly decreasing the amount of purines ingested reduces the substrate for uric acid production.
ii. **Increased Excretion:** Certain foods and ample hydration help the kidneys excrete more uric acid.
iii. **Anti-inflammatory Foods:** Foods rich in antioxidants and anti-inflammatory properties, like berries and leafy greens, can help manage inflammation associated with high uric acid levels.

Evidence Supporting a Low Uric Acid Diet

Numerous studies support the effectiveness of dietary management in controlling uric acid levels:

- **Clinical Trials:** Research shows that reducing purine intake can significantly lower uric acid levels in the blood.
- **Observational Studies:** Populations with diets low in purines, such as certain Mediterranean communities, have lower incidences of gout and kidney stones.

Implementing the Diet

Implementing a low uric acid diet involves:

i. **Meal Planning:** Creating balanced meals that are low in purines and rich in nutrients.
ii. **Grocery Shopping:** Choosing foods that support uric acid management.
iii. **Cooking Methods:** Opting for cooking methods that preserve nutrients and avoid adding unnecessary fats.

4. How to Use This Cookbook

Getting Started

This cookbook is designed to be a comprehensive guide for anyone looking to manage their uric acid levels through diet. Before diving into the recipes, it's essential to understand how to navigate and make the most of this resource.

Understanding the Recipes

Each recipe in this cookbook is carefully crafted to be low in purines while still being delicious and nutritious.

Here's how to approach them:

- **Ingredients List:** Pay attention to the ingredients listed. They are chosen based on their low purine content and health benefits.
- **Serving Sizes:** Proper portion control is crucial. The recipes include recommended serving sizes to help you manage your intake effectively.
- **Nutritional Information:** Each recipe provides detailed nutritional information, including calorie count, macronutrients, and purine content when applicable.

Meal Planning and Preparation

Using this cookbook effectively involves planning and preparation:

- **Weekly Meal Plans:** The cookbook includes sample meal plans to guide you through a balanced week of low uric acid meals. These plans take the guesswork out of daily meal choices and ensure variety and nutritional completeness.
- **Grocery Lists:** Each meal plan is accompanied by a grocery list to streamline your shopping experience. This helps you stay organized and ensures you have all the necessary ingredients on hand.
- **Batch Cooking and Storage Tips:** Many recipes can be prepared in larger quantities and stored for later use. The cookbook provides tips on batch cooking and proper storage methods to save time and reduce food waste.

Adaptation and Personalization

Everyone's dietary needs and preferences are unique. This cookbook offers flexibility and tips for personalization:

- **Dietary Restrictions and Preferences:** Whether you're vegetarian, vegan, gluten-free, or have other dietary restrictions, the cookbook provides modifications and alternative ingredient suggestions to accommodate your needs.
- **Flavor Enhancements:** While keeping purine content low, the recipes include various herbs, spices, and flavorings to ensure meals are tasty and enjoyable.
- **Customization Tips:** Learn how to adapt recipes to better suit your taste preferences or dietary requirements without compromising their low uric acid benefits.

Lifestyle Integration

Integrating a low uric acid diet into your lifestyle involves more than just following recipes:

- **Hydration Reminders:** The importance of hydration is emphasized throughout the cookbook, with reminders and tips for maintaining adequate fluid intake.
- **Physical Activity and Exercise:** The cookbook highlights the role of regular physical activity in managing uric acid levels and provides simple exercise suggestions to complement your dietary efforts.
- **Stress Management:** Recognizing the impact of stress on overall health, the cookbook includes relaxation techniques and stress management tips to support holistic well-being.

Tracking Progress and Staying Motivated

Consistency is key to managing uric acid levels effectively. The cookbook includes tools and strategies to help you stay on track:

- **Food Diary Templates:** Use the provided templates to log your meals, track purine intake, and monitor how different foods affect your uric acid levels.
- **Goal Setting and Reflection:** Set achievable goals for your dietary journey and periodically reflect on your progress. The cookbook offers guidance on setting realistic milestones and celebrating your successes.
- **Troubleshooting Common Challenges:** If you encounter difficulties or setbacks, the cookbook provides troubleshooting tips and solutions to common issues faced during dietary transitions.

Connecting with Support Networks

Building a support system can enhance your success:

- **Family and Friends:** Tips for involving loved ones in your dietary journey, from sharing meals to educating them about your dietary needs.
- **Healthcare Providers:** Guidance on working with healthcare professionals to tailor your diet plan and monitor your uric acid levels.
- **Online Communities:** Suggestions for finding and joining online forums or support groups where you can share experiences, recipes, and encouragement with others on a similar path.

Long-Term Sustainability

The ultimate goal of this cookbook is to help you establish long-term, sustainable dietary habits:

- **Developing a Routine:** Strategies for integrating low uric acid eating habits into your daily life seamlessly.
- **Maintaining Balance:** Tips for balancing your diet with other health considerations, ensuring that you meet all your nutritional needs while keeping uric acid levels in check.
- **Ongoing Education:** Encouragement to stay informed about new research and developments in uric acid management and nutrition.

Conclusion

Using this cookbook as a guide, you can effectively manage your uric acid levels while enjoying delicious, nutritious meals. By understanding the recipes, planning and preparing meals, adapting to your needs, integrating lifestyle changes, tracking progress, connecting with support, and maintaining long-term habits, you'll be well-equipped to achieve and sustain better health.

CHAPTER 1:

FUNDAMENTALS OF A LOW URIC ACID DIET

1.1 Identifying Uric Acid Triggers in Foods

Introduction to Uric Acid Triggers

Understanding the dietary triggers of uric acid is fundamental in managing conditions like gout and hyperuricemia. The foods we consume have a direct impact on the levels of uric acid in our bodies. Certain foods can increase uric acid production, while others can help to reduce it. This section will explore the common dietary culprits that elevate uric acid levels and offer practical advice on how to identify and avoid them.

Purines and Their Role

Purines are natural substances found in many foods. When the body breaks down purines, uric acid is produced as a byproduct. While purines are a necessary part of our DNA and provide important functions, excessive purine intake can lead to high levels of uric acid. Foods high in purines include certain meats, seafood, and alcoholic beverages.

High-Purine Foods

1. **Red Meat**: Beef, pork, and lamb are rich in purines. Organ meats such as liver and kidneys are particularly high in purines and should be avoided by those managing uric acid levels.
2. **Seafood**: Certain fish and shellfish, such as anchovies, sardines, mackerel, and scallops, are high in purines. These should be consumed sparingly or avoided altogether.
3. **Alcohol**: Beer and spirits are significant sources of purines and can lead to increased uric acid production. Beer, in particular, contains yeast, which is high in purines.
4. **Certain Vegetables**: While vegetables generally have lower purine content compared to meats and seafood, some vegetables like asparagus, spinach, and mushrooms do have moderate purine levels.

However, their impact on uric acid levels is less significant than animal-based purines.

Moderate-Purine Foods

While not as high in purines as the foods mentioned above, certain foods still contain moderate amounts of purines and should be eaten in moderation:

- **Poultry**: Chicken and turkey have lower purine levels compared to red meat but should still be consumed in controlled portions.
- **Legumes**: Beans, lentils, and peas have moderate purine content. They can be included in a balanced diet but should not be the primary protein source.
- **Whole Grains**: Foods like oatmeal and bran also contain purines. However, they offer other health benefits and can be consumed in moderation.

Low-Purine Foods

Focusing on low-purine foods is crucial for managing uric acid levels:

- **Fruits**: Most fruits are low in purines and can be consumed freely. Cherries, in particular, have been shown to lower uric acid levels and reduce the risk of gout attacks.
- **Vegetables**: With few exceptions, most vegetables are low in purines. Leafy greens, tomatoes, and bell peppers are excellent choices.
- **Dairy**: Low-fat and non-fat dairy products have been shown to reduce uric acid levels. Milk, yogurt, and cheese are good options.
- **Nuts and Seeds**: These are generally low in purines and provide healthy fats and proteins.

Beverages

- **Water**: Adequate hydration helps the kidneys flush out uric acid. Drinking plenty of water is essential for maintaining healthy uric acid levels.
- **Coffee**: Some studies suggest that coffee may lower uric acid levels and reduce the risk of gout. However, it's best consumed in moderation.

- **Green Tea**: This beverage has been linked to lower uric acid levels due to its antioxidant properties.

Hidden Sources of Purines

- **Processed Foods**: Many processed foods contain additives and preservatives that can increase uric acid production. Always check labels for hidden purine sources.
- **Condiments and Sauces**: Some sauces, especially those made with meat extracts or yeast, can be high in purines.

Practical Tips for Identifying Uric Acid Triggers

1. **Keep a Food Diary**: Tracking what you eat can help identify patterns and foods that trigger uric acid spikes.
2. **Read Labels**: Understanding food labels and ingredient lists can help avoid hidden purines in packaged foods.
3. **Cook at Home**: Preparing meals at home allows you to control ingredients and avoid high-purine foods.
4. **Consult a Dietitian**: A registered dietitian can provide personalized advice and meal plans to help manage uric acid levels effectively.

1.2 Essential Nutrients for Uric Acid Management

Introduction to Nutrient Management

Managing uric acid levels isn't just about avoiding high-purine foods; it's also about ensuring that your diet includes essential nutrients that help in maintaining balanced uric acid levels. Certain nutrients play pivotal roles in reducing uric acid, supporting kidney function, and overall health.

Vitamin C

- **Role in Uric Acid Reduction**: Vitamin C is known to help reduce uric acid levels by enhancing renal function, allowing the kidneys to excrete uric acid more effectively.
- **Sources of Vitamin C**: Citrus fruits (oranges, lemons, grapefruits), strawberries, bell peppers, broccoli, and Brussels sprouts are excellent sources.

- **Daily Intake**: Including a variety of these foods in your daily diet can help ensure adequate vitamin C intake, potentially reducing uric acid levels.

Dairy Products

- **Low-Fat Dairy Benefits**: Studies have shown that low-fat dairy products can lower uric acid levels and decrease the risk of gout.
- **Sources**: Milk, yogurt, and cheese, particularly low-fat or non-fat versions, are beneficial.
- **Daily Recommendations**: Incorporating 2-3 servings of low-fat dairy into your daily diet can be advantageous for managing uric acid levels.

Fiber

- **Role in Uric Acid Management**: Dietary fiber helps in the absorption and elimination of uric acid from the body.
- **Sources of Fiber**: Whole grains (oats, barley, quinoa), fruits (apples, pears, berries), vegetables (carrots, broccoli, beans), and legumes.
- **Daily Intake**: Aim for at least 25-30 grams of fiber daily through a variety of whole foods.

Potassium

- **Kidney Function Support**: Potassium helps in maintaining fluid and electrolyte balance, which is essential for kidney function and uric acid excretion.
- **Sources of Potassium**: Bananas, oranges, potatoes, spinach, and avocados.
- **Daily Recommendations**: Incorporating potassium-rich foods into your diet supports overall kidney health and uric acid management.

Water

- **Hydration and Uric Acid**: Adequate water intake is crucial for diluting uric acid and facilitating its excretion through urine.
- **Daily Recommendations**: Aim to drink at least 8-10 glasses of water daily. Individual needs may vary based on activity level and climate.

Omega-3 Fatty Acids

- **Anti-Inflammatory Properties**: Omega-3 fatty acids help reduce inflammation and may lower the risk of gout attacks.
- **Sources**: Fatty fish (salmon, mackerel, sardines), flaxseeds, chia seeds, and walnuts.
- **Daily Intake**: Including omega-3-rich foods several times a week can support joint health and reduce inflammation.

Antioxidants

- **Role in Uric Acid Management**: Antioxidants help neutralize free radicals and reduce oxidative stress, which can contribute to lower uric acid levels.
- **Sources of Antioxidants**: Berries (blueberries, strawberries, raspberries), nuts (almonds, pecans), and green leafy vegetables.
- **Daily Recommendations**: A diet rich in a variety of colorful fruits and vegetables ensures a good intake of antioxidants.

Cherries

- **Special Role in Gout Management**: Cherries, particularly tart cherries, have been shown to lower uric acid levels and reduce the frequency of gout attacks.
- **Consumption**: Fresh, dried, or in juice form, cherries can be a beneficial addition to your diet.
- **Daily Intake**: Incorporating a handful of cherries or a glass of cherry juice daily can have positive effects on uric acid levels.

Magnesium

- **Uric Acid Excretion**: Magnesium plays a role in the excretion of uric acid and can help prevent its crystallization.
- **Sources of Magnesium**: Nuts (almonds, cashews), seeds (pumpkin seeds, sunflower seeds), leafy greens (spinach, Swiss chard), and whole grains.
- **Daily Recommendations**: Including a variety of magnesium-rich foods in your diet supports uric acid management and overall health.

In conclusion, Incorporating essential nutrients into your diet is a proactive approach to managing uric acid levels and preventing related health issues. By focusing on foods rich in vitamin C, fiber, potassium, omega-3 fatty acids, antioxidants, and specific beneficial foods like low-fat dairy and cherries, you can effectively support your body's natural ability to manage and excrete uric acid. Ensuring adequate hydration and including a diverse range of nutrient-dense foods will contribute to overall health and well-being, while also keeping uric acid levels in check.

Practical Tips for Incorporating Essential Nutrients

1. **Variety is Key**: Eating a wide range of foods ensures you get a mix of essential nutrients. Aim to include different fruits, vegetables, grains, and proteins in your meals.
2. **Meal Planning**: Plan your meals and snacks to include nutrient-rich foods. For instance, have a citrus fruit with breakfast, a salad with leafy greens for lunch, and a serving of fish or dairy at dinner.
3. **Healthy Snacks**: Choose nutrient-dense snacks like fruit, nuts, yogurt, and vegetable sticks to help meet your daily nutrient requirements.
4. **Stay Hydrated**: Carry a water bottle with you to ensure you are drinking enough water throughout the day. Herbal teas and water-rich fruits and vegetables can also contribute to your fluid intake.
5. **Cooking Methods**: Opt for cooking methods that preserve nutrients, such as steaming, grilling, or baking, rather than frying. Avoid overcooking vegetables to retain their vitamin content.
6. **Reading Food Labels**: Pay attention to food labels to ensure you are choosing products that are low in added sugars, sodium, and unhealthy fats, and high in beneficial nutrients.
7. **Supplements**: If you find it challenging to get certain nutrients from food alone, consider discussing supplementation with your healthcare provider.

Monitoring and Adjusting Your Diet

Regularly reviewing your diet and its effects on your health can help in making necessary adjustments. Keeping a food diary can be a valuable tool for tracking what you eat and identifying any areas that need improvement. Additionally, regular check-ups with your healthcare provider can help monitor your uric acid levels and overall health, providing guidance on any dietary changes needed.

1.3 The Importance of Portion Control

Introduction to Portion Control

Portion control plays a vital role in managing uric acid levels and maintaining overall health. Overeating, even healthy foods, can lead to weight gain and increased uric acid production. By understanding and practicing portion control, you can ensure that you consume the right amount of food for your body's needs without overloading it with purines or calories.

Why Portion Control Matters

1. **Calorie Management**: Consuming too many calories can lead to weight gain, which is a risk factor for increased uric acid levels and gout. Maintaining a healthy weight through portion control can help reduce these risks.
2. **Balanced Nutrient Intake**: Portion control helps ensure you get a balanced intake of nutrients without overconsuming any one food group. This balance is essential for overall health and effective uric acid management.
3. **Preventing Overeating**: Large portions can lead to overeating, even when the food is healthy. Overeating puts a strain on the digestive system and can lead to the overproduction of uric acid.
4. **Mindful Eating**: Practicing portion control encourages mindful eating, which helps you pay attention to hunger and fullness cues, making it easier to avoid overeating.

How to Practice Portion Control

1. **Understanding Serving Sizes**: Familiarize yourself with standard serving sizes for different food groups. For example, a serving of meat is typically 3-4 ounces, a serving of fruits or vegetables is about one cup, and a serving of grains is one-half cup cooked.
2. **Using Smaller Plates**: Eating from smaller plates can help control portions by making smaller amounts of food appear more substantial. This psychological trick can help reduce the tendency to overeat.
3. **Measuring Portions**: Use measuring cups, spoons, and a kitchen scale to measure your food portions, especially when starting. This practice helps you get a better understanding of what appropriate portion sizes look like.
4. **Serving and Storing Food**: Serve food in individual portions rather than from large, communal dishes to avoid the temptation of second helpings. Store leftovers in portion-sized containers for easy future meals.
5. **Eating Slowly**: Take your time to eat and chew your food thoroughly. Eating slowly allows your brain to register fullness, helping to prevent overeating.
6. **Avoiding Distractions**: Eating without distractions, such as television or mobile phones, helps you focus on your food and recognize when you are full.

Specific Strategies for Different Meals

- **Breakfast**: Start the day with a balanced meal that includes protein, fiber, and healthy fats. For example, a serving of oatmeal with fruit and a small amount of nuts can provide sustained energy.
- **Lunch**: Opt for a combination of lean protein, whole grains, and vegetables. A typical portion might include a 3-ounce piece of grilled chicken, one cup of quinoa, and a side salad.
- **Dinner**: Keep dinner portions moderate. Focus on filling half your plate with vegetables, one-quarter with lean protein, and one-quarter with whole grains.
- **Snacks**: Choose nutrient-dense snacks like a piece of fruit, a handful of nuts, or yogurt. Measure out single servings to avoid mindless snacking.

Dealing with Eating Out

1. **Restaurant Portions**: Restaurant portions are often larger than necessary. Consider splitting a meal with a friend, ordering a half portion, or taking half of your meal home.
2. **Healthy Choices**: Choose dishes that are grilled, steamed, or baked instead of fried. Opt for vegetables or salad as side dishes rather than high-purine foods like fries or heavy sauces.
3. **Controlling Sauces and Dressings**: Ask for sauces and dressings on the side to control how much you use. This practice can significantly reduce calorie and purine intake.
4. **Mindful Eating**: Even when eating out, practice mindful eating by taking your time to savor your food and paying attention to your hunger and fullness cues.

Portion Control and Specific Dietary Needs

- **Vegetarian and Vegan Diets**: Ensure you are getting enough protein from plant-based sources like beans, lentils, and tofu, but be mindful of their purine content and portion sizes.
- **Low-Carb Diets**: Focus on high-quality protein and healthy fats while managing portion sizes to avoid overconsumption.
- **Mediterranean Diet**: Emphasize fruits, vegetables, whole grains, and healthy fats like olive oil, but pay attention to portion sizes to maintain balance.

1.4 Reading Food Labels and Ingredients

Introduction to Food Labels

Reading food labels is an essential skill for anyone managing their diet, particularly for those focused on controlling uric acid levels. Food labels provide valuable information about the nutritional content of products, helping you make informed choices about what to eat. Understanding how to read and interpret these labels can aid in selecting foods that are low in purines and supportive of overall health.

Components of a Food Label

- **Serving Size**: The serving size indicates the amount of food that the nutritional information pertains to. It's important to compare this with the actual amount you eat to understand your intake accurately.
- **Calories**: This section shows the number of calories per serving. Monitoring calorie intake helps in managing weight, which is crucial for controlling uric acid levels.
- **Nutrient Breakdown**: This includes information on macronutrients (carbohydrates, proteins, fats) and micronutrients (vitamins and minerals).
- **Ingredients List**: Ingredients are listed in descending order by weight. The first few ingredients make up the bulk of the product.
- **Percent Daily Values (%DV)**: These values indicate how much a nutrient in a serving of food contributes to a daily diet, based on a 2,000-calorie per day intake.

Understanding Nutrient Information

- **Total Fat, Saturated Fat, and Trans Fat**: High intake of unhealthy fats can contribute to weight gain and increased uric acid levels. Look for products with low amounts of saturated and trans fats.
- **Cholesterol**: High dietary cholesterol can also impact uric acid levels and overall heart health. Choose foods with lower cholesterol content.
- **Sodium**: Excess sodium can lead to water retention and increased blood pressure, which is important to manage for overall health. Opt for products with lower sodium levels.
- **Carbohydrates**: Includes total carbs, dietary fiber, and sugars. Focus on high-fiber foods, as fiber helps in managing uric acid levels.
- **Protein**: While protein is essential, be mindful of the source. Opt for low-purine protein sources like dairy, eggs, and plant-based proteins.

- **Vitamins and Minerals**: Ensure you are getting sufficient vitamins and minerals like vitamin C, potassium, and magnesium, which help in uric acid management.

Identifying Hidden Purines

- **Meat Extracts and Broths**: These can be hidden sources of purines. Look for terms like "meat extract," "beef broth," "chicken stock," and "bone broth" on the ingredients list, as these can be high in purines and should be consumed in moderation.
- **Yeast Extracts**: Common in processed foods, yeast extracts like Marmite and Vegemite are high in purines. Ingredients such as "autolyzed yeast extract" and "hydrolyzed yeast" are also worth noting.
- **Certain Condiments and Sauces**: Some condiments, especially those containing anchovies or other fish products (like Worcestershire sauce and some salad dressings), can add hidden purines to your diet.
- **Processed and Pre-Packaged Foods**: These often contain additives and preservatives that might contribute to uric acid levels. Always check for hidden ingredients that may not be immediately obvious as purine sources.

Label Claims and What They Mean

- **"Low Fat"**: Indicates that the product contains 3 grams or less of fat per serving. While good for overall health, it's essential to check the rest of the nutritional information to ensure it's low in other areas like purines and sodium.
- **"Low Sodium"**: Contains 140 milligrams or less of sodium per serving. Beneficial for overall health, especially for individuals managing blood pressure.
- **"No Added Sugars"**: No sugars were added during processing, but naturally occurring sugars may still be present. Helpful for reducing calorie intake and managing weight.
- **"Whole Grain"**: The product contains 100% whole grains, which are high in fiber and beneficial for managing uric acid levels.

- **"High in Fiber"**: Contains 5 grams or more of fiber per serving. High-fiber foods aid in digestion and can help manage uric acid levels.
- **"Organic"**: Indicates that the food was produced without synthetic pesticides, GMOs, or artificial additives. While this can be better for overall health, it does not necessarily mean it's low in purines or beneficial for uric acid management.

Using the Information

- **Compare Products**: Use the nutritional labels to compare different brands and choose the one with the lowest purine content, lower unhealthy fats, and higher beneficial nutrients.
- **Plan Your Meals**: Incorporate label reading into your meal planning. For example, if choosing a canned soup, opt for one with lower sodium and no meat extracts.
- **Cooking from Scratch**: Whenever possible, cook meals from scratch using fresh ingredients. This allows full control over what goes into your food, helping to avoid hidden purines and excess sodium.
- **Portion Awareness**: Be mindful of the serving size listed on the label. If you consume more than the serving size, adjust the nutritional values accordingly to reflect your actual intake.

Tips for Shopping

- **Shop the Perimeter**: Most supermarkets are arranged with fresh produce, meats, dairy, and bakery items around the perimeter. These fresh foods are typically lower in purines and higher in essential nutrients.
- **Check for Hidden Ingredients**: Processed foods in the center aisles can contain hidden purines and other additives. Always read labels carefully before purchasing.
- **Whole Foods Focus**: Prioritize whole foods like fresh fruits, vegetables, whole grains, and lean proteins. These are less likely to contain hidden purines and are better for overall health.

- **Stay Informed**: Keep up to date with food labeling regulations and changes. This knowledge helps in making informed choices at the grocery store.

In summary, the fundamentals of a low uric acid diet encompass understanding and identifying uric acid triggers in foods, incorporating essential nutrients for uric acid management, practicing portion control, and mastering the skill of reading food labels and ingredients. Each of these elements plays a crucial role in effectively managing uric acid levels and preventing related health issues such as gout.

CHAPTER 2:

MEAL PLANNING AND PREPARATION

2.1 Building a Weekly Low Uric Acid Meal Plan

Introduction to Meal Planning

Creating a weekly meal plan is an essential step for anyone managing uric acid levels. A well-thought-out plan helps ensure you are eating a balanced diet that supports your health goals, avoids high-purine foods, and includes essential nutrients. Meal planning not only simplifies grocery shopping but also makes it easier to stick to a low uric acid diet.

Benefits of Meal Planning

- **Consistency**: Regularly eating meals that are low in purines helps maintain stable uric acid levels.
- **Variety**: Planning in advance allows you to incorporate a variety of foods and nutrients, preventing monotony.
- **Cost-Efficiency**: Planning helps avoid last-minute takeout and reduces food waste, saving money.
- **Time Management**: Having a plan reduces the time spent deciding what to eat each day and ensures you always have the ingredients you need.

Steps to Build a Weekly Meal Plan

- **Assess Your Dietary Needs**: Understand your specific dietary requirements. Consult with a healthcare provider to get a clear idea of your caloric needs, nutritional goals, and any specific foods to avoid.

- **Research Low Purine Foods**: Make a list of low purine foods that you enjoy. Common low purine foods include most fruits, vegetables, whole grains, low-fat dairy, and nuts.
- **Create a Template**: Design a weekly meal plan template that includes breakfast, lunch, dinner, and snacks. This helps visualize your meals for the week.
- **Balance Your Meals**: Ensure each meal includes a balance of protein, carbohydrates, and fats. For example, a balanced breakfast could include oatmeal (carbohydrate), a small serving of nuts (fat), and a piece of fruit (fiber and vitamins).
- **Incorporate Variety**: Rotate different proteins, vegetables, and grains throughout the week to keep meals interesting and nutritionally diverse.

Tips for Effective Meal Planning

- **Prep Ingredients**: Prepare ingredients in advance to save time during the week. Chop vegetables, cook grains, and portion out snacks on a dedicated meal prep day.
- **Batch Cooking**: Cook larger quantities of staple foods (like quinoa, brown rice, and roasted vegetables) and use them in different meals throughout the week.
- **Flexible Recipes**: Choose recipes that are easy to modify based on what you have on hand. For example, a stir-fry can incorporate any combination of vegetables you have available.
- **Seasonal Produce**: Use seasonal produce to ensure freshness and cost-effectiveness. Seasonal fruits and vegetables are often more affordable and nutritious.
- **Stay Hydrated**: Include beverages like water, herbal teas, and low-sugar drinks in your meal plan to stay hydrated.

Adjusting Your Meal Plan

Regularly review and adjust your meal plan based on your preferences and nutritional needs. It's important to keep track of how your body responds to different foods and make adjustments as necessary. Flexibility is key to maintaining a sustainable meal planning routine.

In conclusion, building a weekly low uric acid meal plan is a practical and effective way to manage your diet and support your health. By focusing on low purine foods, balancing nutrients, and incorporating variety, you can create a meal plan that is both enjoyable and beneficial for managing uric acid levels. Consistent meal planning not only simplifies your daily routine but also ensures you are taking proactive steps towards better health.

2.2 Smart Grocery Shopping Strategies

Introduction to Smart Grocery Shopping

Smart grocery shopping is crucial for maintaining a low uric acid diet. Making informed choices at the grocery store can help you avoid high-purine foods and ensure you have the ingredients needed for healthy, balanced meals. By developing effective shopping strategies, you can save time, money, and effort while sticking to your dietary goals.

Preparing for Your Shopping Trip

- **Create a Shopping List**: Start by making a detailed shopping list based on your weekly meal plan. Organize the list by sections of the store to streamline your shopping experience.
- **Check Inventory**: Before heading to the store, check your kitchen inventory to avoid buying items you already have. This helps reduce waste and saves money.
- **Plan Your Budget**: Set a budget for your grocery trip to manage expenses. Knowing your budget helps you make cost-effective choices without compromising on quality.
- **Eat Before Shopping**: Avoid grocery shopping on an empty stomach. Being hungry can lead to impulse buying, often resulting in unhealthy choices.

Navigating the Grocery Store

- **Shop the Perimeter**: Focus on the store's perimeter where fresh produce, dairy, and meats are usually located. These areas are less likely to have processed foods that may contain hidden purines.
- **Read Labels**: Take the time to read food labels carefully. Look for hidden purines, added sugars, sodium, and unhealthy fats. Opt for whole foods with minimal ingredients.
- **Buy Seasonal and Local**: Seasonal and locally sourced produce is often fresher, more nutritious, and more affordable. Check for local farmers' markets or the seasonal section of your grocery store.
- **Choose Whole Grains**: When selecting grains, choose whole grain options like brown rice, quinoa, and whole wheat products. These are higher in fiber and nutrients.

Selecting Specific Food Groups

- **Fruits and Vegetables**: Fill your cart with a variety of colorful fruits and vegetables. Aim for at least five servings of fruits and vegetables each day, focusing on low-purine options.
- **Proteins**: Choose lean proteins like chicken, turkey, fish, and plant-based proteins such as beans, lentils, and tofu. Avoid high-purine meats like organ meats and certain seafood.
- **Dairy**: Select low-fat or non-fat dairy products, which are lower in purines and beneficial for uric acid management. Options include milk, yogurt, and cheese.
- **Beverages**: Opt for water, herbal teas, and low-sugar drinks. Avoid sugary sodas and alcohol, which can increase uric acid levels.

Cost-Saving Strategies

- **Buy in Bulk**: Purchase staple items like grains, beans, and nuts in bulk to save money. Ensure proper storage to maintain freshness.
- **Use Coupons and Discounts**: Take advantage of coupons, store discounts, and loyalty programs to reduce costs.

- **Compare Prices**: Compare prices between different brands and stores to find the best deals. Generic or store brands can often be as good as name brands at a lower cost.
- **Plan for Leftovers**: Cook larger portions of meals that can be used as leftovers. This reduces the need for additional cooking and minimizes food waste.

Online Grocery Shopping

- **Convenience**: Online grocery shopping can save time and make it easier to stick to your list without the temptation of impulse buys.
- **Price Comparison**: Online shopping allows for easy comparison of prices and finding the best deals.
- **Delivery Options**: Many online grocery stores offer delivery services, which can be especially useful for those with busy schedules.
- **Review Products**: Take advantage of product reviews and ratings to make informed choices about the quality and taste of items.

Environmental Considerations

- **Reusable Bags**: Bring reusable shopping bags to reduce plastic waste. Many stores offer discounts for using your bags.
- **Eco-Friendly Products**: Choose products with minimal packaging or environmentally friendly packaging materials.
- **Local and Sustainable**: Support local farmers and producers who use sustainable farming practices. This not only benefits the environment but also supports the local economy.

In summary, smart grocery shopping strategies are essential for maintaining a low uric acid diet and overall health. By preparing a detailed shopping list, navigating the store efficiently, selecting nutrient-rich foods, and using cost-saving techniques, you can ensure your kitchen is stocked with ingredients that support your dietary goals. Making informed choices at the grocery store lays the foundation for successful meal planning and healthy eating habits.

2.3 Time-Saving Meal Prep Techniques

Introduction to Meal Prep

Meal prepping involves preparing meals or meal components in advance to save time and ensure you have healthy options readily available. For those managing uric acid levels, meal prepping can be a game-changer, helping you stay on track with your dietary goals and reduce the stress of daily cooking.

Benefits of Meal Prep

- **Consistency**: Having prepped meals on hand ensures you consistently consume low-purine foods, which helps maintain stable uric acid levels.
- **Stress Reduction**: Knowing that meals are ready to go reduces the daily stress of deciding what to cook and helps avoid last-minute unhealthy choices.
- **Portion Control**: Prepping meals in advance allows you to portion out servings correctly, which is crucial for managing weight and nutrient intake.
- **Cost Efficiency**: Buying ingredients in bulk and preparing them at home can save money compared to eating out or buying pre-packaged meals.
- **Waste Reduction**: Meal prepping helps minimize food waste by using up all the ingredients you buy and ensuring leftovers are consumed.

Steps for Effective Meal Prep

1. **Plan Your Meals**: Start by planning your meals for the week. Consider breakfast, lunch, dinner, and snacks. Use your weekly meal plan as a guide.
2. **Make a Shopping List**: Create a detailed shopping list based on your meal plan. This ensures you have all the necessary ingredients and helps you avoid impulse purchases.

3. **Designate Prep Time**: Set aside a specific time each week dedicated to meal prepping. Many people find that spending a few hours on a weekend works best.
4. **Organize Your Kitchen**: Make sure your kitchen is clean and organized before you start prepping. Have containers, utensils, and appliances ready to use.

Techniques for Efficient Meal Prep

1. **Batch Cooking**: Cook large quantities of staple foods like grains, proteins, and vegetables that can be used in various meals throughout the week. For example, cook a large pot of quinoa, roast several trays of vegetables, and grill chicken breasts.
2. **One-Pot Meals**: Prepare one-pot meals such as soups, stews, and casseroles that can be portioned out and reheated easily. These meals often taste better as leftovers since flavors have more time to meld.
3. **Freezing Portions**: Freeze individual portions of meals that can be thawed and eaten later. This is especially useful for nights when you don't have time to cook.
4. **Ingredient Prep**: Prepare ingredients in advance to make assembling meals quicker. Chop vegetables, marinate proteins, and portion out snacks.

Storage Tips

- **Use Clear Containers**: Store prepped food in clear containers so you can easily see what you have. Glass containers are a good option as they are microwave safe and don't retain odors.
- **Label and Date**: Label each container with the contents and the date it was prepared. This helps keep track of freshness and ensures you use up older items first.
- **Proper Refrigeration and Freezing**: Make sure to store prepped meals and ingredients in the fridge or freezer at the appropriate temperature to maintain freshness and prevent spoilage.
- **Healthy Meal Prep Recipes**

Staying Motivated

- **Track Your Progress**: Keep a meal prep journal to track your meals, note what worked well, and make adjustments for future weeks.
- **Involve the Family**: Get family members involved in meal prepping. This can make the process more enjoyable and ensures everyone is on board with the meal plan.
- **Experiment with New Recipes**: Keep meal prep interesting by trying new recipes and incorporating different flavors and cuisines.

Time-saving meal prep techniques are invaluable for anyone managing uric acid levels and aiming to maintain a healthy diet. By dedicating time to prepare meals and ingredients in advance, you can ensure consistent consumption of low-purine foods, reduce daily stress, and make healthy eating more convenient. With effective planning, batch cooking, and proper storage, meal prepping can become a seamless part of your routine, supporting your dietary goals and overall well-being.

2.4 Stocking Your Kitchen with Essentials

Introduction to Kitchen Essentials

Stocking your kitchen with the right essentials is a key component of maintaining a low uric acid diet. Having the necessary tools, ingredients, and appliances on hand makes meal preparation easier, more efficient, and more enjoyable.

Essential Kitchen Tools and Equipment

- **Cutting Boards**: Invest in several cutting boards to prevent cross-contamination between raw meats and vegetables. Choose boards that are durable and easy to clean.
- **Knives**: A good set of knives, including a chef's knife, paring knife, and serrated knife, is essential for efficient food preparation.
- **Pots and Pans**: A variety of pots and pans, including a large stockpot, sauté pan, and non-stick skillet, are necessary for cooking a range of dishes.

- **Measuring Cups and Spoons**: Accurate measuring tools are crucial for following recipes and controlling portion sizes.
- **Mixing Bowls**: A set of mixing bowls in various sizes is useful for preparing ingredients and mixing recipes.
- **Blender/Food Processor**: These appliances are invaluable for making smoothies, soups, sauces, and more.
- **Baking Sheets and Dishes**: Have a few baking sheets and casserole dishes for roasting vegetables, baking proteins, and preparing casseroles.
- **Storage Containers**: Invest in high-quality storage containers for storing prepped meals and leftovers. Choose containers that are microwave and dishwasher safe.

Staple Ingredients for a Low Uric Acid Diet

1. **Fruits and Vegetables**: Stock a variety of fresh, frozen, and canned fruits and vegetables. Opt for low-purine choices like berries, apples, bananas, leafy greens, and bell peppers.
2. **Whole Grains**: Keep whole grains like brown rice, quinoa, oats, and whole wheat pasta on hand. These are high in fiber and beneficial for managing uric acid levels.
3. **Lean Proteins**: Include lean protein sources such as chicken, turkey, tofu, beans, and lentils in your kitchen. Avoid high-purine meats and organ meats.
4. **Low-Fat Dairy**: Stock low-fat or non-fat dairy products like milk, yogurt, and cheese. These are good sources of calcium and protein.
5. **Healthy Fats**: Include healthy fats like olive oil, avocado oil, nuts, and seeds. These provide essential fatty acids and support overall health.
6. **Spices and Herbs**: Keep a variety of spices and herbs to add flavor to your meals without extra salt or fat. Common choices include garlic powder, onion powder, basil, oregano, and cumin.
7. **Condiments**: Choose condiments that are low in added sugars and sodium. Look for mustard, vinegar, low-sodium soy sauce, and salsa.

Organizing Your Kitchen

- **Pantry Organization**: Arrange your pantry so that frequently used items are easily accessible. Use clear containers to store dry goods and label everything for quick identification.
- **Refrigerator and Freezer Organization**: Keep your refrigerator and freezer organized by grouping items by category (e.g., dairy, proteins, vegetables) and using clear containers or bins to separate different types of food. This helps prevent food from getting lost or forgotten and makes it easier to see what you have on hand.
- **Refrigerator Essentials**
- **Fresh Produce**: Store a variety of fresh fruits and vegetables in the crisper drawers. Leafy greens, berries, apples, and bell peppers are great low-purine options.
- **Lean Proteins**: Keep lean proteins like chicken breasts, turkey slices, tofu, and low-fat dairy products in the main compartments.
- **Condiments and Dressings**: Choose low-sodium and low-sugar options for condiments. Store items like mustard, vinegar, salsa, and homemade dressings on the refrigerator door.
- **Prepared Foods**: Store prepped meals and leftovers in clear, airtight containers. Label and date them to keep track of freshness.

Freezer Essentials

- **Frozen Vegetables and Fruits**: Keep a variety of frozen vegetables and fruits on hand for quick meals and smoothies. Frozen produce retains most of its nutritional value and is convenient for meal prep.
- **Lean Proteins**: Stock up on lean proteins like chicken, fish, and tofu. Portion them out and freeze in individual servings for easy thawing and cooking.
- **Whole Grains**: Cook and freeze portions of whole grains like quinoa, brown rice, and barley. These can be quickly reheated for meals.
- **Prepared Meals**: Batch cook meals and freeze portions for future use. This is especially useful for busy days when you don't have time to cook from scratch.

Pantry Essentials

- **Whole Grains and Legumes**: Keep a variety of whole grains (e.g., brown rice, quinoa, oats) and legumes (e.g., lentils, black beans, chickpeas) in your pantry. These are versatile and form the basis of many low-purine meals.
- **Canned Goods**: Stock canned vegetables, beans, and low-sodium broths. These are convenient for quick meals and add variety to your diet.
- **Nuts and Seeds**: Store a selection of nuts and seeds (e.g., almonds, walnuts, chia seeds) for healthy snacks and toppings. Choose unsalted and raw options when possible.
- **Oils and Vinegars**: Keep healthy oils (e.g., olive oil, avocado oil) and a variety of vinegars (e.g., apple cider vinegar, balsamic vinegar) for cooking and dressings.
- **Spices and Herbs**: Stock a range of spices and dried herbs to add flavor to your meals. Common choices include garlic powder, cumin, basil, oregano, and paprika.

Maintaining a Stocked Kitchen

- **Regular Inventory Checks**: Periodically check your pantry, fridge, and freezer to see what needs to be replenished. Keeping a running list of items to restock helps prevent running out of essentials.
- **Rotation System**: Use a first-in, first-out (FIFO) system to ensure older items are used before newer ones. This helps reduce food waste and keeps ingredients fresh.
- **Bulk Purchases**: Buy non-perishable items in bulk to save money. Store them properly to maintain their quality and shelf life.
- **Emergency Staples**: Keep a small supply of emergency staples like canned beans, pasta, and rice. These can be lifesavers on days when you need a quick meal.

Adapting Your Kitchen for a Low Uric Acid Diet

1. **Focus on Fresh and Whole Foods**: Prioritize fresh and whole foods over processed items. Fresh produce, lean proteins, and whole grains should be the foundation of your diet.

2. **Avoid High-Purine Foods**: Be mindful of foods high in purines and avoid stocking them in your kitchen. Common high-purine foods include red meat, organ meats, certain seafood (e.g., anchovies, sardines), and high-fructose corn syrup.
3. **Hydration Options**: Keep your kitchen stocked with plenty of hydration options. Water, herbal teas, and low-sugar beverages are ideal. Avoid sugary sodas and excessive alcohol, as they can increase uric acid levels.
4. **Healthy Snack Choices**: Choose healthy snack options like fruits, vegetables, nuts, and yogurt. Avoid snacks that are high in sugar, salt, and unhealthy fats.

In conclusion, stocking your kitchen with the right essentials is a critical step in maintaining a low uric acid diet. Having the necessary tools, ingredients, and equipment on hand makes meal preparation easier, more efficient, and more enjoyable. By organizing your kitchen, focusing on fresh and whole foods, and regularly checking your inventory, you can ensure that your kitchen supports your dietary goals and overall health. With a well-stocked kitchen, you'll be better equipped to prepare healthy, low-purine meals that help manage your uric acid levels and promote a balanced, nutritious diet.

CHAPTER 3:

LIFESTYLE AND DIETARY ADJUSTMENTS

3.1 Hydration and Its Impact on Uric Acid Levels

Understanding Uric Acid and Its Importance

Uric acid is a natural waste product formed during the breakdown of purines, substances found in many foods and human cells. Normally, uric acid dissolves in the blood and is excreted through the kidneys in urine. However, elevated levels can lead to crystallization in joints, causing gout— a painful form of arthritis.

Hydration and Uric Acid Levels

Hydration plays a crucial role in managing uric acid levels. When you're well-hydrated, your kidneys function more efficiently, flushing out excess uric acid before it can crystallize. Studies have shown that maintaining adequate hydration helps reduce the risk of gout attacks and may even lower uric acid levels over time.

Recommended Fluid Intake

The recommended fluid intake varies depending on individual factors such as age, gender, health status, and climate. Generally, aiming for at least 8 glasses (about 2 liters) of water per day is a good starting point. However, this can vary; some individuals may need more, especially if they are physically active or live in hot climates.

Impact of Different Fluids

Not all fluids are equal when it comes to managing uric acid levels. Water is the best choice because it contains no purines or added sugars, both of which can contribute to uric acid production. Sugary drinks and alcohol, on the other hand, have been linked to increased uric acid levels and should be consumed in moderation or avoided.

Hydration Tips

To ensure optimal hydration:

- **Drink Water Regularly:** Sip water throughout the day rather than consuming large amounts at once.
- **Monitor Urine Color:** Pale yellow urine usually indicates adequate hydration.
- **Consider Electrolytes:** In cases of prolonged physical activity or sweating, electrolyte-rich fluids or sports drinks can help maintain hydration balance.

In conclusion, adequate hydration is crucial for managing uric acid levels. By maintaining proper fluid intake, primarily through water consumption, individuals can support kidney function and reduce the risk of gout attacks.

3.2 The Role of Physical Activity in Uric Acid Management

Introduction to Physical Activity and Uric Acid

Physical activity plays a significant role in overall health, including its impact on uric acid levels and gout management. Understanding how exercise influences uric acid metabolism can guide individuals in making informed decisions about their physical fitness routines.

Mechanisms Behind Exercise and Uric Acid Levels

- **Increased Uric Acid Excretion:** Exercise stimulates blood flow and kidney function, which can enhance the excretion of uric acid through urine. This helps prevent uric acid from accumulating in joints and tissues.
- **Weight Management:** Regular physical activity contributes to weight loss or maintenance. Excess body weight is a risk factor for hyperuricemia (elevated uric acid levels), so maintaining a healthy weight through exercise can lower the risk of gout attacks.

- **Improvement in Insulin Sensitivity:** Some studies suggest that exercise improves insulin sensitivity, which may indirectly affect uric acid metabolism since insulin resistance is associated with higher uric acid levels.

Types of Exercise Beneficial for Uric Acid Management

1. **Aerobic Exercises:** Activities like walking, jogging, swimming, and cycling are effective in improving cardiovascular health and promoting uric acid excretion.
2. **Resistance Training:** Strength training exercises, such as weightlifting or resistance band workouts, help build muscle mass and support weight management, which can indirectly benefit uric acid levels.
3. **Flexibility and Balance Exercises:** While not directly affecting uric acid metabolism, these exercises contribute to overall physical well-being, which is essential for maintaining an active lifestyle.

Exercise Recommendations

The American College of Sports Medicine (ACSM) recommends:

- **150 minutes of moderate-intensity aerobic exercise** per week, or 75 minutes of vigorous-intensity exercise spread throughout the week.
- **Strength training exercises** targeting major muscle groups on two or more days per week.

Individuals with gout or elevated uric acid levels should start gradually and consult with healthcare professionals to tailor exercise programs to their specific needs and abilities.

Considerations and Precautions

- **Hydration:** Maintain adequate fluid intake during exercise to support kidney function and prevent dehydration, which can potentially elevate uric acid levels.

- **Joint Health:** Choose low-impact exercises if joints are affected by gout to minimize discomfort and reduce the risk of exacerbating symptoms.
- **Medication Adjustment:** Some medications used to manage gout may interact with exercise or require adjustments. Consult healthcare providers for guidance.

In summary, regular physical activity is an integral part of managing uric acid levels and reducing the risk of gout attacks. By promoting uric acid excretion, supporting weight management, and improving overall health, exercise contributes positively to gout management strategies.

3.3 Stress Reduction Techniques

Understanding the Impact of Stress on Uric Acid Levels

Stress is a common factor in modern lifestyles and can significantly affect overall health, including uric acid levels. When stressed, the body releases hormones like cortisol, which can lead to increased uric acid production and decreased excretion, potentially exacerbating gout symptoms.

Effective Stress Reduction Techniques

Mindfulness Meditation:

- **Technique:** Mindfulness meditation involves focusing on the present moment without judgment, which can reduce stress levels and promote relaxation.
- **Benefits:** Studies suggest that regular practice of mindfulness meditation may lower cortisol levels, thereby potentially reducing uric acid production associated with stress.

Yoga:

- **Technique:** Yoga combines physical postures, breathing exercises, and meditation techniques to promote physical and mental well-being.

- **Benefits:** Yoga has been shown to lower cortisol levels, improve mood, and reduce perceived stress, which can indirectly support uric acid management.

Deep Breathing Exercises:
- **Technique:** Deep breathing exercises, such as diaphragmatic breathing or belly breathing, involve taking slow, deep breaths to activate the body's relaxation response.
- **Benefits:** These exercises help calm the nervous system, reduce stress hormones like cortisol, and promote relaxation, which can help stabilize uric acid levels.

Physical Activity:
- **Technique:** Regular aerobic exercise and physical activity not only improve physical health but also release endorphins, the body's natural mood elevators.
- **Benefits:** Exercise reduces stress, improves sleep quality, and enhances overall well-being, all of which contribute to better stress management and potentially lower uric acid levels.

Social Support:
- **Technique:** Maintaining strong social connections and seeking support from friends, family, or support groups can help reduce feelings of stress and anxiety.
- **Benefits:** Having a support network provides emotional reassurance, practical help, and a sense of belonging, which can buffer the impact of stress on uric acid levels.

Lifestyle Modifications for Stress Reduction

Healthy Sleep Habits:
- **Technique:** Establishing a consistent sleep routine, practicing good sleep hygiene, and ensuring adequate sleep duration (7-9 hours per night for adults) are crucial for stress management and overall health.
- **Benefits:** Quality sleep supports hormone regulation, including cortisol levels, and promotes optimal physical and mental functioning.

Balanced Nutrition:
- **Technique:** Adopting a balanced diet rich in fruits, vegetables, whole grains, lean proteins, and healthy fats supports overall health and may mitigate the impact of stress on uric acid levels.
- **Benefits:** Nutrient-dense foods provide essential vitamins and minerals that support stress resilience and overall well-being.

Incorporating Stress Reduction Techniques into Daily Life
- **Consistency:** Engage in stress reduction techniques regularly to build resilience and maintain lower stress levels over time.
- **Personalization:** Experiment with different techniques to find what works best for individual preferences and lifestyle.
- **Professional Guidance:** Consider consulting healthcare professionals or stress management specialists for personalized recommendations and support.

Effective stress reduction techniques, such as mindfulness meditation, yoga, deep breathing exercises, physical activity, and social support, play a crucial role in managing stress levels and potentially mitigating the impact on uric acid levels. By incorporating these techniques into daily routines, individuals can enhance overall well-being and support their gout management strategies.

3.4 Tracking Your Progress and Making Adjustments

Importance of Tracking
Tracking your progress is essential in any health-related endeavor, including managing uric acid levels and implementing lifestyle changes. It provides valuable insights into the effectiveness of your strategies and allows for timely adjustments to optimize outcomes.

Methods of Tracking
Symptom Diary:

- **Purpose:** Keep a daily or weekly record of gout symptoms, including pain intensity, swelling, and affected joints.
- **Benefits:** Helps identify triggers or patterns related to uric acid fluctuations, guiding dietary and lifestyle adjustments.

Uric Acid Levels:

- **Testing:** Regular monitoring of uric acid levels through blood tests, typically recommended every 3-6 months or as advised by healthcare providers.
- **Benefits:** Provides quantitative data on uric acid levels, assessing the effectiveness of interventions and guiding treatment decisions.

Lifestyle Habits:

- **Daily Log:** Maintain a journal of hydration levels, dietary intake (including purine-rich foods and alcohol consumption), exercise routines, stress levels, and sleep patterns.
- **Benefits:** Helps identify correlations between lifestyle habits and uric acid levels, facilitating targeted adjustments.

Setting Goals

SMART Goals:

- **Specific:** Clearly define what you aim to achieve, such as reducing uric acid levels by a certain amount or decreasing the frequency of gout attacks.
- **Measurable:** Use quantifiable metrics, such as uric acid levels or symptom frequency, to track progress.
- **Achievable:** Set realistic goals that align with your health status, lifestyle, and medical recommendations.
- **Relevant:** Ensure goals are meaningful and directly contribute to improving uric acid management and overall health.
- **Time-bound:** Establish a timeline for achieving goals, creating accountability and motivation.

Long-Term vs. Short-Term Goals:

- **Long-Term:** Focus on sustainable lifestyle changes, such as maintaining a healthy diet and regular exercise routine.
- **Short-Term:** Set incremental goals, such as reducing intake of purine-rich foods or increasing water consumption, to achieve long-term objectives.

Analyzing Progress
Regular Reviews:

- **Frequency:** Schedule regular reviews of your tracking data, such as weekly or monthly, to assess progress and identify trends.
- **Reflection:** Reflect on achievements, challenges encountered, and adjustments made to refine your approach.

Consultation with Healthcare Providers:

- **Collaboration:** Share tracking data with healthcare providers during appointments to evaluate effectiveness of interventions and make informed decisions.
- **Guidance:** Seek guidance on interpreting data, adjusting treatment plans, and addressing any concerns or challenges.

Making Adjustments
Evidence-Based Adjustments:

- **Data-Informed Decisions:** Use tracking data to identify areas needing improvement and implement evidence-based adjustments.
- **Iterative Process:** Adjust interventions, such as modifying diet, exercise routines, stress management techniques, or medication, based on outcomes and new information.

Seeking Support:

- **Healthcare Team:** Collaborate with healthcare providers, including doctors, dietitians, and specialists, for personalized guidance and support.
- **Peer Support:** Engage with support groups or online communities to share experiences, gain insights, and stay motivated.

In conclusion, tracking your progress in managing uric acid levels through methods such as symptom diaries, uric acid level monitoring, and lifestyle habit logs is crucial for evaluating effectiveness, setting goals, and making informed adjustments. By adopting a systematic approach to tracking and analyzing data, individuals can optimize their gout management strategies and improve overall health outcomes.

CHAPTER 4:

ADAPTING TO DIFFERENT SCENARIOS

4.1 Eating Out While Maintaining a Low Uric Acid Diet

Introduction to Eating Out and Uric Acid Management
Eating out can present challenges for those managing uric acid levels, as restaurant meals often contain ingredients high in purines or other substances that can trigger gout attacks. However, with careful planning and awareness, it's possible to enjoy dining out while maintaining a low uric acid diet.

Understanding Purine Content in Restaurant Foods
Common Culprits:
- **Meat and Seafood:** Dishes like steak, organ meats (liver, kidneys), shellfish (shrimp, lobster), and gravies are high in purines.
- **Alcohol:** Beer and certain spirits can raise uric acid levels.
- **Processed Foods:** Items like processed meats (sausages, hot dogs) and high-fat dishes may also contribute to uric acid production.

Healthy Choices:
- **Vegetarian Options:** Plant-based dishes like salads, vegetable stir-fries, or bean-based meals are generally lower in purines.

- **Lean Proteins:** Opt for grilled or baked lean meats like chicken or turkey breast instead of red meat or fatty cuts.

Strategies for Eating Out with a Low Uric Acid Diet
Menu Research:

- **Preparation:** Before dining out, check the restaurant's menu online if available. Look for dishes that align with a low purine diet.
- **Customization:** Don't hesitate to ask for modifications, such as requesting grilled instead of fried, or sauces and dressings on the side to control portion size and purine intake.

Portion Control:

- **Sharing:** Consider sharing larger portions or appetizers with others to manage portion sizes and reduce purine intake.
- **Avoid Buffets:** Buffets can be tempting, but they often offer high-purine choices in abundance.

Dining Tips for Specific Types of Cuisine
Asian Cuisine:

- **Options:** Choose stir-fried or steamed dishes with vegetables and lean proteins. Avoid deep-fried or heavily sauced items.
- **Soy Sauce:** Use low-sodium soy sauce sparingly, as it can be high in salt and may affect uric acid levels.

Italian Cuisine:

- **Choices:** Opt for pasta with tomato-based sauces rather than creamy or meat-based sauces. Select pizzas with vegetable toppings and minimal cheese.
- **Moderation:** Enjoy bread in moderation, as it can contribute to higher uric acid levels.

Managing Alcohol Consumption

- **Selection:** If consuming alcohol, opt for options like wine or spirits in moderation rather than beer, which is high in purines.

- **Hydration:** Drink plenty of water alongside alcohol to help flush out uric acid and stay hydrated.

In conclusion, eating out while maintaining a low uric acid diet requires careful planning and smart choices. By researching menus, choosing wisely, and controlling portion sizes, individuals can enjoy dining out without compromising their gout management efforts.

4.2 Travel Tips for Staying on Track

Traveling can disrupt routine and pose challenges for individuals managing uric acid levels. Changes in diet, hydration, and activity levels during travel can impact uric acid metabolism and increase the risk of gout attacks. However, with preparation and awareness, it's possible to maintain a low uric acid diet and stay on track while traveling.

Planning Ahead for Travel
Research Destination:
- **Culinary Culture:** Understand typical local dishes and ingredients. Research restaurants or grocery stores that offer options aligned with a low purine diet.
- **Medical Supplies:** Pack necessary medications and supplements prescribed for gout management.
- **Meal Preparation:**
- **Snacks:** Pack healthy snacks like fruits, nuts, or low-purine protein bars to avoid relying on high-purine airport or roadside options.
- **Meal Substitutes:** Consider carrying meal substitutes like instant oatmeal packets or protein shakes for quick and nutritious alternatives.

Making Smart Food Choices While Traveling
Airport and Roadside Stops:

- **Options:** Look for salads, sandwiches with lean meats, or grilled chicken options at airport cafes or fast-food outlets.
- **Avoidance:** Steer clear of deep-fried foods, processed snacks, and sugary beverages that can contribute to uric acid buildup.

Hotel Accommodations:

- **Requesting Amenities:** Choose accommodations with kitchenettes or request a mini-fridge to store fresh produce and prepare simple meals.
- **Breakfast Options:** Opt for oatmeal, yogurt, fresh fruits, and whole-grain cereals during hotel breakfasts to start the day with low-purine choices.

Dining Strategies During Travel
Local Cuisine Exploration:

- **Adaptation:** Seek out restaurants offering grilled or steamed dishes, seafood without rich sauces, and vegetable-based meals typical of the local diet.
- **Communication:** Communicate dietary preferences and restrictions clearly to restaurant staff to ensure meals are prepared accordingly.
- **Hydration Management:**
- **Water Intake:** Carry a reusable water bottle and stay hydrated throughout travel to support kidney function and uric acid excretion.
- **Limit Alcohol:** Minimize alcohol intake during travel, as it can dehydrate the body and elevate uric acid levels.

Handling Time Zone Changes and Jet Lag
Adjusting Meal Times:

- **Gradual Transition:** Gradually adjust meal times to align with local schedules to minimize disruptions to digestion and metabolic processes.
- **Healthy Choices:** Choose light and easily digestible meals upon arrival to ease the transition and avoid exacerbating gout symptoms.

Emergency Preparedness

- **Medical Assistance:** Identify nearby medical facilities or pharmacies at your travel destination in case of gout flare-ups or medication needs.
- **Insurance Coverage:** Ensure travel insurance covers medical emergencies, including gout-related incidents, for peace of mind during international travel.

In summary, traveling while managing uric acid levels requires proactive planning and mindful choices. By researching destinations, preparing meals and snacks, making smart food choices, and staying hydrated, individuals can maintain a low uric acid diet and minimize the risk of gout attacks while enjoying their travels.

4.3 Special Considerations for Different Dietary Preferences

Managing uric acid levels involves understanding how different dietary preferences can impact purine intake and overall health. Whether following vegetarian, vegan, or other specific diets, individuals can adapt their eating habits to support gout management effectively.

Vegetarian and Vegan Diets
Purine Sources in Plant-Based Foods:
- **Legumes:** Beans, lentils, and peas are high in purines but can still be part of a balanced diet.
- **Vegetables:** Some vegetables like spinach, mushrooms, and asparagus contain moderate levels of purines.
- **Moderation:** While plant-based diets generally have lower purine content than animal-based diets, specific food choices and portion sizes still matter.

Balancing Protein Intake:
- **Sources:** Include a variety of plant-based proteins such as tofu, tempeh, quinoa, and nuts to meet protein needs without excessive purine intake.

- **Supplementation:** Consider vitamin B12 and iron supplementation, as vegan diets may require additional attention to nutrient intake.

Mediterranean Diet
Overview:
- **Principles:** Emphasizes fruits, vegetables, whole grains, legumes, nuts, seeds, and olive oil, with moderate intake of fish, poultry, and dairy.
- **Impact on Uric Acid:** The Mediterranean diet is generally associated with lower inflammation and improved heart health, potentially beneficial for managing gout.

Moderating Red Meat and Alcohol:
- **Limitations:** Red meat and alcohol consumption, even in moderation, should be monitored due to their potential to raise uric acid levels.

Low-Carb and Keto Diets
Focus on Protein and Fats:
- **Purine Sources:** Diets high in animal proteins and fats may increase uric acid levels, potentially triggering gout attacks.
- **Balancing Act:** Incorporate low-purine vegetables, healthy fats like avocados, and lean proteins to maintain a balanced approach.

Hydration and Electrolytes:
- **Importance:** Ensure adequate hydration and electrolyte balance, especially during the initial stages of ketogenic diet adaptation, to support kidney function and minimize uric acid buildup.

Gluten-Free Diet
Potential Challenges:
- **Processed Foods:** Some gluten-free products may contain higher levels of refined carbohydrates and additives, which can impact uric acid levels.
- **Whole Foods:** Emphasize naturally gluten-free foods like fruits, vegetables, lean proteins, and gluten-free grains to maintain a balanced diet.

Personalized Dietary Approaches
Consultation with Healthcare Providers:
- **Individualized Guidance:** Seek advice from healthcare providers or registered dietitians to tailor dietary recommendations based on personal health needs and preferences.
- **Monitoring:** Regularly monitor uric acid levels and gout symptoms to assess the impact of dietary changes and make necessary adjustments.

In summary, managing uric acid levels effectively involves adapting dietary preferences to minimize purine intake while supporting overall health and nutritional needs. Whether following vegetarian, Mediterranean, low-carb, or other specialized diets, individuals can make informed choices to support gout management and improve overall well-being.

CHAPTER 5:

HEALTHY, NUTRICIOUS, AND DELICIOUS LOW URIC ACID DIET RECIPES

5.1 Breakfast Recipes

1. Oatmeal with Fresh Berries and Almonds
Intro: Oatmeal with fresh berries and almonds is a nutritious and filling breakfast that provides a great start to your day. Packed with fiber, antioxidants, and healthy fats, this dish helps in maintaining stable energy levels and supports uric acid management.

Total Prep Time
- 15 minutes

Ingredients
- 1 cup rolled oats
- 2 cups water or unsweetened almond milk
- 1/2 cup fresh berries (blueberries, strawberries, raspberries)
- 1/4 cup sliced almonds

- 1 tablespoon honey or maple syrup (optional)
- 1/2 teaspoon cinnamon (optional)

Instructions

1. In a medium saucepan, bring water or almond milk to a boil.
2. Add the rolled oats and reduce the heat to a simmer. Cook for about 5-7 minutes, stirring occasionally, until the oats are soft and have absorbed most of the liquid.
3. Remove from heat and let it sit for a couple of minutes to thicken.
4. Transfer the oatmeal to a bowl and top with fresh berries and sliced almonds.
5. Drizzle with honey or maple syrup and sprinkle with cinnamon, if desired.
6. Serve warm.

Nutritional Information (per serving)

- Calories: 320
- Protein: 8g
- Carbohydrates: 45g
- Fiber: 8g
- Fat: 12g

Tips for Making it Low Uric Acid-Friendly

- Use unsweetened almond milk instead of dairy milk to reduce purine intake.
- Choose a variety of fresh berries for their antioxidant properties and low purine content.
- Avoid adding too much sweetener; the natural sweetness of berries is often sufficient.

2. Spinach and Mushroom Egg White Omelette

Intro: This spinach and mushroom egg white omelette is a light and protein-packed breakfast option that's perfect for those managing their uric acid levels. The inclusion of vegetables adds fiber and essential nutrients to your meal.

Total Prep Time

- 20 minutes

Ingredients

- 4 egg whites
- 1 cup fresh spinach, chopped
- 1/2 cup mushrooms, sliced
- 1 small onion, finely chopped
- 1 tablespoon olive oil
- Salt and pepper to taste

Instructions

1. Heat olive oil in a non-stick skillet over medium heat.
2. Add onions and mushrooms to the skillet and sauté until they are soft and the mushrooms release their moisture.
3. Add the spinach and cook until wilted, then remove the vegetables from the skillet and set aside.
4. In a bowl, whisk the egg whites with a pinch of salt and pepper.
5. Pour the egg whites into the skillet and cook until they start to set.
6. Spread the sautéed vegetables evenly over one half of the omelette.
7. Carefully fold the other half of the omelette over the vegetables and cook for another minute.
8. Slide the omelette onto a plate and serve hot.

Nutritional Information (per serving)

- Calories: 120
- Protein: 15g
- Carbohydrates: 5g
- Fiber: 2g
- Fat: 5g

Tips for Making it Low Uric Acid-Friendly

- Use egg whites only, as the yolks contain higher amounts of purines.
- Incorporate a variety of low-purine vegetables like spinach and mushrooms.
- Cook with olive oil, which is a healthy fat that supports overall health.

3. Whole Grain Toast with Avocado and Tomato

Intro: Whole grain toast with avocado and tomato is a simple yet delicious breakfast option that combines the healthy fats of avocado with the fiber of whole grain bread and the freshness of tomatoes.

Total Prep Time

- 10 minutes

Ingredients

- 2 slices whole grain bread
- 1 ripe avocado
- 1 medium tomato, sliced
- Salt and pepper to taste
- Lemon juice (optional)
- Fresh basil or cilantro for garnish (optional)

Instructions

1. Toast the whole grain bread slices to your desired level of crispiness.
2. While the bread is toasting, cut the avocado in half, remove the pit, and scoop the flesh into a bowl. Mash the avocado with a fork until smooth.
3. Spread the mashed avocado evenly over the toasted bread slices.
4. Top with tomato slices and season with salt and pepper.
5. Drizzle with a bit of lemon juice for added flavor, if desired.
6. Garnish with fresh basil or cilantro and serve immediately.

Nutritional Information (per serving)

- Calories: 250
- Protein: 6g
- Carbohydrates: 28g
- Fiber: 8g
- Fat: 15g

Tips for Making it Low Uric Acid-Friendly

- Choose whole grain bread to increase fiber intake, which can help with digestion and overall health.
- Avocado is a great source of healthy fats and is low in purines.

- Tomatoes add a fresh, low-purine component that enhances the meal's flavor.

4. Greek Yogurt with Honey and Walnuts

Intro: Greek yogurt with honey and walnuts is a protein-rich breakfast that's easy to prepare and offers a perfect balance of sweetness and crunch. This combination is also packed with probiotics and healthy fats.

Total Prep Time

- 5 minutes

Ingredients

- 1 cup plain Greek yogurt
- 1 tablespoon honey
- 2 tablespoons chopped walnuts
- 1/2 teaspoon vanilla extract (optional)

Instructions

1. Scoop the Greek yogurt into a bowl.
2. Drizzle the honey over the yogurt.
3. Sprinkle with chopped walnuts.
4. Add vanilla extract for extra flavor, if desired.
5. Stir gently and enjoy immediately.

Nutritional Information (per serving)

- Calories: 250
- Protein: 15g
- Carbohydrates: 20g
- Fiber: 2g
- Fat: 10g

Tips for Making it Low Uric Acid-Friendly

- Use plain Greek yogurt, as it's lower in sugar and additives.
- Honey is a natural sweetener that should be used in moderation.
- Walnuts provide healthy fats and are low in purines, making them a suitable choice for this diet.

5. Banana and Blueberry Smoothie Bowl

Intro: The banana and blueberry smoothie bowl is a vibrant and refreshing breakfast that combines the natural sweetness of fruits with the creaminess of yogurt. It's a nutrient-dense way to start your day.

Total Prep Time

- 10 minutes

Ingredients

- 1 frozen banana
- 1/2 cup fresh or frozen blueberries
- 1/2 cup plain Greek yogurt
- 1/4 cup unsweetened almond milk
- 1 tablespoon chia seeds
- Toppings: sliced banana, fresh blueberries, granola, shredded coconut

Instructions

1. In a blender, combine the frozen banana, blueberries, Greek yogurt, almond milk, and chia seeds. Blend until smooth.
2. Pour the smoothie into a bowl.
3. Top with sliced banana, fresh blueberries, granola, and shredded coconut.
4. Serve immediately.

Nutritional Information (per serving)

- Calories: 350
- Protein: 12g
- Carbohydrates: 60g
- Fiber: 10g
- Fat: 8g

Tips for Making it Low Uric Acid-Friendly

- Use plain Greek yogurt and unsweetened almond milk to keep added sugars low.
- Incorporate a variety of fruits, but focus on those lower in purines like bananas and blueberries.
- Add chia seeds for extra fiber and omega-3 fatty acids.

6. Quinoa Breakfast Porridge with Almond Milk

Intro: Quinoa breakfast porridge with almond milk is a wholesome and protein-packed alternative to traditional oatmeal. This dish is rich in essential amino acids and provides a hearty start to your morning.

Total Prep Time

- 20 minutes

Ingredients

- 1 cup quinoa, rinsed
- 2 cups unsweetened almond milk
- 1 tablespoon maple syrup or honey
- 1 teaspoon vanilla extract
- Toppings: fresh berries, chopped nuts, sliced banana

Instructions

1. In a medium saucepan, combine the quinoa and almond milk. Bring to a boil over medium heat.
2. Reduce the heat to low and simmer, covered, for about 15 minutes or until the quinoa is tender and the milk is mostly absorbed.
3. Stir in the maple syrup or honey and vanilla extract.
4. Divide the porridge into bowls and top with fresh berries, chopped nuts, and sliced banana.
5. Serve warm.

Nutritional Information (per serving)

- Calories: 300
- Protein: 8g
- Carbohydrates: 50g
- Fiber: 5g
- Fat: 8g

Tips for Making it Low Uric Acid-Friendly

- Use almond milk to keep the dish dairy-free and lower in purines.
- Incorporate a variety of fruits and nuts for added nutrients and flavor.
- Choose natural sweeteners like honey or maple syrup in moderation.

7. Apple Cinnamon Overnight Oats

Intro: Apple cinnamon overnight oats are a convenient and nutritious breakfast option that can be prepared the night before. This dish combines the comforting flavors of apple and cinnamon with the health benefits of oats.

Total Prep Time

- 10 minutes (plus overnight chilling)

Ingredients

- 1 cup rolled oats
- 1 cup unsweetened almond milk
- 1/2 cup plain Greek yogurt
- 1 apple, diced
- 1 tablespoon chia seeds
- 1 teaspoon cinnamon
- 1 tablespoon honey or maple syrup (optional)

Instructions

1. In a bowl or jar, combine the rolled oats, almond milk, Greek yogurt, diced apple, chia seeds, and cinnamon. Stir well to combine.
2. If desired, add honey or maple syrup for sweetness and stir again.
3. Cover the bowl or jar with a lid or plastic wrap and refrigerate overnight.
4. In the morning, give the oats a good stir and add a splash of almond milk if needed to adjust the consistency.
5. Serve chilled, topped with additional apple slices or nuts if desired.

Nutritional Information (per serving)

- Calories: 350
- Protein: 12g
- Carbohydrates: 55g
- Fiber: 8g
- Fat: 8g

Tips for Making it Low Uric Acid-Friendly

- Use unsweetened almond milk to keep the dish dairy-free.
- Incorporate a variety of fruits like apples which are low in purines.
- Choose natural sweeteners like honey or maple syrup in moderation.

8. Chia Seed Pudding with Mixed Fruits

Intro: Chia seed pudding with mixed fruits is a delicious and nutritious breakfast that's rich in fiber, omega-3 fatty acids, and antioxidants. This easy-to-make dish is perfect for a healthy start to your day.

Total Prep Time
- 10 minutes (plus overnight chilling)

Ingredients
- 1/4 cup chia seeds
- 1 cup unsweetened almond milk
- 1 tablespoon honey or maple syrup
- 1/2 teaspoon vanilla extract
- Mixed fruits (e.g., berries, kiwi, mango)

Instructions
1. In a bowl or jar, combine the chia seeds, almond milk, honey or maple syrup, and vanilla extract. Stir well to combine.
2. Cover and refrigerate for at least 4 hours, or overnight, until the chia seeds have absorbed the liquid and the mixture has thickened.
3. Before serving, give the pudding a good stir.
4. Top with mixed fruits and serve chilled.

Nutritional Information (per serving)
- Calories: 200
- Protein: 5g
- Carbohydrates: 30g
- Fiber: 10g
- Fat: 8g

Tips for Making it Low Uric Acid-Friendly
- Use unsweetened almond milk to keep the dish dairy-free.

- Incorporate a variety of low-purine fruits like berries, kiwi, and mango.
- Opt for natural sweeteners like honey or maple syrup in moderation.

9. Scrambled Tofu with Vegetables

Intro: Scrambled tofu with vegetables is a plant-based breakfast that's packed with protein and nutrients. It's a flavorful and satisfying way to start your day, especially for those looking to avoid animal products.

Total Prep Time

- 20 minutes

Ingredients

- 1 block firm tofu, drained and crumbled
- 1 tablespoon olive oil
- 1 small onion, finely chopped
- 1 bell pepper, diced
- 1 cup spinach, chopped
- 1/2 cup cherry tomatoes, halved
- 1/2 teaspoon turmeric
- Salt and pepper to taste

Instructions

1. Heat olive oil in a skillet over medium heat.
2. Add the chopped onion and bell pepper, and sauté until they are soft.
3. Add the crumbled tofu to the skillet and stir well.
4. Sprinkle turmeric over the tofu and mix until evenly coated.
5. Add the spinach and cherry tomatoes to the skillet and cook until the spinach is wilted and the tomatoes are soft.
6. Season with salt and pepper to taste.
7. Serve hot.

Nutritional Information (per serving)

- Calories: 220
- Protein: 15g
- Carbohydrates: 10g
- Fiber: 4g

- Fat: 14g

Tips for Making it Low Uric Acid-Friendly
- Use firm tofu as a low-purine protein source.
- Include a variety of low-purine vegetables like spinach, bell pepper, and tomatoes.
- Cook with olive oil, which is a healthy fat.

10. Whole Wheat Pancakes with Maple Syrup

Intro: Whole wheat pancakes with maple syrup are a delicious and healthier alternative to traditional pancakes. They are made with whole grain flour, providing more fiber and nutrients.

Total Prep Time
- 30 minutes

Ingredients
- 1 cup whole wheat flour
- 1 tablespoon baking powder
- 1 tablespoon sugar
- 1/2 teaspoon salt
- 1 cup unsweetened almond milk
- 1 large egg
- 1 tablespoon olive oil
- Maple syrup for serving

Instructions
1. In a large bowl, whisk together the whole wheat flour, baking powder, sugar, and salt.
2. In another bowl, combine the almond milk, egg, and olive oil.
3. Pour the wet ingredients into the dry ingredients and stir until just combined.
4. Heat a non-stick skillet over medium heat and lightly grease with a small amount of olive oil.
5. Pour 1/4 cup of batter onto the skillet for each pancake.
6. Cook until bubbles form on the surface of the pancakes, then flip and cook until golden brown on the other side.

7. Serve warm with maple syrup.

Nutritional Information (per serving)

- Calories: 200
- Protein: 5g
- Carbohydrates: 35g
- Fiber: 5g
- Fat: 5g

Tips for Making it Low Uric Acid-Friendly

- Use whole wheat flour to increase fiber and nutrient content.
- Opt for unsweetened almond milk to keep the recipe dairy-free.
- Use maple syrup in moderation as a natural sweetener.

11. Baked Sweet Potato and Black Bean Hash

Intro: Baked sweet potato and black bean hash is a hearty and flavorful breakfast that combines the sweetness of sweet potatoes with the savory taste of black beans. It's a nutrient-dense meal that's perfect for starting your day.

Total Prep Time

- 45 minutes

Ingredients

1. 2 large sweet potatoes, peeled and diced
2. 1 can black beans, drained and rinsed
3. 1 bell pepper, diced
4. 1 small onion, chopped
5. 2 tablespoons olive oil
6. 1 teaspoon cumin
7. 1/2 teaspoon smoked paprika
8. Salt and pepper to taste
9. Fresh cilantro for garnish

Instructions

1. Preheat your oven to 400°F (200°C).
2. In a large bowl, combine the diced sweet potatoes, black beans, bell pepper, and onion.

3. Drizzle with olive oil and sprinkle with cumin, smoked paprika, salt, and pepper. Toss to coat.
4. Spread the mixture in a single layer on a baking sheet.
5. Bake for 30-35 minutes, stirring halfway through, until the sweet potatoes are tender and lightly browned.
6. Garnish with fresh cilantro and serve hot.

Nutritional Information (per serving)
- Calories: 350
- Protein: 8g
- Carbohydrates: 65g
- Fiber: 12g
- Fat: 10g

Tips for Making it Low Uric Acid-Friendly
- Sweet potatoes are low in purines and provide a good source of vitamins and fiber.
- Black beans are a healthy plant-based protein option.
- Use olive oil for cooking, which is beneficial for overall health.

12. Green Smoothie with Spinach, Kale, and Pineapple

Intro: A green smoothie with spinach, kale, and pineapple is a refreshing and nutrient-packed drink that's perfect for a quick and healthy breakfast. It's rich in vitamins, minerals, and antioxidants.

Total Prep Time
- 10 minutes

Ingredients
- 1 cup fresh spinach
- 1/2 cup fresh kale, stems removed
- 1 cup pineapple chunks (fresh or frozen)
- 1 banana
- 1 cup unsweetened almond milk
- 1 tablespoon chia seeds (optional)

Instructions
1. Add the spinach, kale, pineapple chunks, banana, and almond milk to a blender.

2. Blend until smooth and creamy.
3. If desired, add chia seeds and blend for a few more seconds.
4. Pour into a glass and serve immediately.

Nutritional Information (per serving)

- Calories: 180
- Protein: 3g
- Carbohydrates: 35g
- Fiber: 6g
- Fat: 3g

Tips for Making it Low Uric Acid-Friendly

- Use a variety of low-purine greens like spinach and kale.
- Pineapple adds natural sweetness without high purine content.
- Almond milk keeps the smoothie dairy-free and low in purines.

13. Buckwheat Pancakes with Fresh Berries

Intro: Buckwheat pancakes with fresh berries are a gluten-free and nutrient-dense breakfast option. Buckwheat flour provides a rich source of fiber and essential nutrients, making these pancakes both delicious and healthy.

Total Prep Time

- 30 minutes

Ingredients

- 1 cup buckwheat flour
- 1 tablespoon baking powder
- 1 tablespoon sugar
- 1/2 teaspoon salt
- 1 cup unsweetened almond milk
- 1 large egg
- 1 tablespoon olive oil
- Fresh berries for topping
- Maple syrup for serving

Instructions

1. In a large bowl, whisk together the buckwheat flour, baking powder, sugar, and salt.
2. In another bowl, combine the almond milk, egg, and olive oil.
3. Pour the wet ingredients into the dry ingredients and stir until just combined.
4. Heat a non-stick skillet over medium heat and lightly grease with a small amount of olive oil.
5. Pour 1/4 cup of batter onto the skillet for each pancake.
6. Cook until bubbles form on the surface of the pancakes, then flip and cook until golden brown on the other side.
7. Serve warm with fresh berries and a drizzle of maple syrup.

Nutritional Information (per serving)
- Calories: 210
- Protein: 6g
- Carbohydrates: 40g
- Fiber: 5g
- Fat: 5g

Tips for Making it Low Uric Acid-Friendly
- Buckwheat flour is a great gluten-free alternative and low in purines.
- Use unsweetened almond milk to keep the dish dairy-free.
- Top with fresh berries for added vitamins, antioxidants, and natural sweetness.

14. Cottage Cheese with Fresh Peaches

Intro: Cottage cheese with fresh peaches is a quick and nutritious breakfast that combines the creamy texture of cottage cheese with the juicy sweetness of peaches. It's a high-protein option that's easy to prepare.

Total Prep Time
- 5 minutes

Ingredients
- 1 cup low-fat cottage cheese
- 1 ripe peach, sliced

- 1 tablespoon honey (optional)
- Fresh mint for garnish (optional)

Instructions

1. Scoop the cottage cheese into a bowl.
2. Top with sliced peaches.
3. Drizzle with honey if desired.
4. Garnish with fresh mint and serve immediately.

Nutritional Information (per serving)

- Calories: 180
- Protein: 14g
- Carbohydrates: 20g
- Fiber: 2g
- Fat: 5g

Tips for Making it Low Uric Acid-Friendly

- Choose low-fat cottage cheese to reduce overall fat intake.
- Use fresh peaches which are low in purines and add natural sweetness.
- Opt for honey in moderation if you need additional sweetness.

15. Almond Butter and Banana on Whole Grain Toast

Intro: Almond butter and banana on whole grain toast is a delicious and filling breakfast that provides a perfect balance of carbohydrates, healthy fats, and protein. It's quick to make and very satisfying.

Total Prep Time

- 5 minutes

Ingredients

- 2 slices whole grain bread
- 2 tablespoons almond butter
- 1 banana, sliced
- A pinch of cinnamon (optional)

Instructions

1. Toast the whole grain bread slices to your desired level of crispiness.
2. Spread almond butter evenly on each slice of toast.

3. Top with banana slices.
4. Sprinkle with a pinch of cinnamon if desired.
5. Serve immediately.

Nutritional Information (per serving)

- Calories: 300
- Protein: 8g
- Carbohydrates: 40g
- Fiber: 8g
- Fat: 12g

Tips for Making it Low Uric Acid-Friendly

- Use whole grain bread to increase fiber intake.
- Almond butter provides healthy fats and protein without high purine content.
- Bananas are low in purines and add natural sweetness.

16. Herbed Greek Yogurt with Cucumber and Tomato Salad

Intro: Herbed Greek yogurt with cucumber and tomato salad is a refreshing and protein-rich breakfast option. The combination of creamy yogurt and fresh vegetables makes for a nutritious and tasty meal.

Total Prep Time

- 15 minutes

Ingredients

- 1 cup plain Greek yogurt
- 1/2 cucumber, diced
- 1 cup cherry tomatoes, halved
- 2 tablespoons fresh dill, chopped
- 1 tablespoon fresh mint, chopped
- 1 tablespoon lemon juice
- Salt and pepper to taste

Instructions

1. In a bowl, combine the Greek yogurt, cucumber, cherry tomatoes, dill, and mint.
2. Stir in the lemon juice and season with salt and pepper to taste.
3. Mix well and serve immediately.

Nutritional Information (per serving)

- Calories: 150
- Protein: 10g
- Carbohydrates: 10g
- Fiber: 2g
- Fat: 8g

Tips for Making it Low Uric Acid -Friendly

- Use plain Greek yogurt for its high protein and probiotic benefits.
- Incorporate fresh vegetables like cucumber and tomatoes, which are low in purines.
- Herbs add flavor without the need for excessive salt or high-purine ingredients.

17. Poached Eggs on Whole Grain English Muffin

Intro: Poached eggs on a whole grain English muffin is a classic breakfast that's high in protein and fiber. It's simple to make and provides a nutritious start to your day.

Total Prep Time

- 20 minutes

Ingredients

- 2 large eggs
- 1 whole grain English muffin, split and toasted
- 1 teaspoon vinegar
- Salt and pepper to taste
- Fresh herbs for garnish (optional)

Instructions

1. Bring a pot of water to a gentle simmer and add the vinegar.
2. Crack each egg into a small bowl and gently slide them into the simmering water.

3. Poach the eggs for about 3-4 minutes, until the whites are set but the yolks are still runny.
4. Remove the eggs with a slotted spoon and drain on paper towels.
5. Place the poached eggs on the toasted English muffin halves.
6. Season with salt and pepper and garnish with fresh herbs if desired.
7. Serve immediately.

Nutritional Information (per serving)
- Calories: 250
- Protein: 15g
- Carbohydrates: 25g
- Fiber: 5g
- Fat: 10g

Tips for Making it Low Uric Acid-Friendly
- Choose whole grain English muffins to increase fiber content.
- Poaching eggs instead of frying reduces added fats.
- Garnish with fresh herbs to add flavor without adding purines.

18. Homemade Granola with Dried Fruits

Intro: Homemade granola with dried fruits is a crunchy and delicious breakfast that you can prepare in advance. It's perfect for pairing with yogurt or milk and provides a healthy mix of oats, nuts, and fruits.

Total Prep Time
- 40 minutes

Ingredients
- 3 cups rolled oats
- 1 cup nuts (almonds, walnuts, or pecans)
- 1/2 cup honey or maple syrup
- 1/4 cup olive oil
- 1 teaspoon vanilla extract
- 1 cup dried fruits (raisins, cranberries, apricots)
- 1 teaspoon cinnamon (optional)

Instructions

1. Preheat your oven to 300°F (150°C).
2. In a large bowl, combine the rolled oats and nuts.
3. In a small saucepan, heat the honey or maple syrup, olive oil, and vanilla extract until combined. Pour over the oats and nuts and mix well.
4. Spread the mixture on a baking sheet lined with parchment paper.
5. Bake for 25-30 minutes, stirring every 10 minutes, until the granola is golden brown.
6. Remove from the oven and stir in the dried fruits.
7. Allow the granola to cool completely before storing in an airtight container.

Nutritional Information (per serving)

- Calories: 250
- Protein: 6g
- Carbohydrates: 35g
- Fiber: 5g
- Fat: 10g

Tips for Making it Low Uric Acid-Friendly

- Use a variety of nuts and dried fruits that are low in purines.
- Opt for natural sweeteners like honey or maple syrup in moderation.
- Pair with low-fat yogurt or almond milk for a balanced meal.

19. Pumpkin Spice Oatmeal

Intro: Pumpkin spice oatmeal is a comforting and flavorful breakfast that's perfect for the fall season. Made with real pumpkin and warming spices, it's a nutritious and delicious way to start your day.

Total Prep Time

- 15 minutes

Ingredients

- 1 cup rolled oats
- 2 cups water or unsweetened almond milk
- 1/2 cup pumpkin puree

- 1 tablespoon maple syrup
- 1 teaspoon pumpkin pie spice
- 1/4 teaspoon vanilla extract
- Toppings: chopped nuts, dried cranberries

Instructions

1. In a medium saucepan, bring water or almond milk to a boil.
2. Add the rolled oats and reduce the heat to a simmer. Cook for about 5-7 minutes, stirring occasionally, until the oats are soft and have absorbed most of the liquid.
3. Stir in the pumpkin puree, maple syrup, pumpkin pie spice, and vanilla extract.
4. Cook for an additional 2-3 minutes until heated through.
5. Serve warm with your favorite toppings.

Nutritional Information (per serving)

- Calories: 250
- Protein: 6g
- Carbohydrates: 45g
- Fiber: 7g
- Fat: 5g

Tips for Making it Low Uric Acid-Friendly

- Use unsweetened almond milk to keep the dish dairy-free.
- Incorporate pumpkin puree for added vitamins and fiber.
- Opt for natural sweeteners like maple syrup in moderation.

20. Spinach and Feta Stuffed Whole Grain Crepes

Intro: Spinach and feta stuffed whole grain crepes are a savory and nutritious breakfast option that's perfect for a special morning. The combination of whole grains, fresh spinach, and tangy feta creates a delightful meal.

Total Prep Time

- 45 minutes

Ingredients

- 1 cup whole grain flour

- 1 1/4 cups unsweetened almond milk
- 2 large eggs
- 1 tablespoon olive oil
- 1/2 teaspoon salt
- 1 cup fresh spinach, chopped
- 1/2 cup feta cheese, crumbled
- 1 small onion, finely chopped
- 1 tablespoon olive oil (for filling)

Instructions

1. In a bowl, whisk together the whole grain flour, almond milk, eggs, olive oil, and salt until smooth. Let the batter rest for 30 minutes.
2. Heat a non-stick skillet over medium heat and lightly grease with a small amount of olive oil.
3. Pour about 1/4 cup of the batter into the skillet, tilting the pan to spread the batter evenly.
4. Cook for about 1-2 minutes, until the edges start to lift and the crepe is lightly browned on the bottom. Flip and cook for another 1-2 minutes. Repeat with the remaining batter.
5. In another skillet, heat 1 tablespoon of olive oil over medium heat.
6. Add the chopped onion and sauté until soft and translucent.
7. Add the spinach and cook until wilted.
8. Remove from heat and stir in the feta cheese.
9. Place a spoonful of the spinach and feta mixture on one half of each crepe.
10. Fold the crepe over the filling and serve warm.

Nutritional Information (per serving)

- Calories: 300
- Protein: 12g
- Carbohydrates: 35g
- Fiber: 5g
- Fat: 12g

Tips for Making it Low Uric Acid-Friendly

- Use whole grain flour for added fiber and nutrients.

- Incorporate fresh spinach, which is low in purines and high in vitamins.
- Use feta cheese in moderation to avoid excessive dairy intake.

These recipes are designed to provide a variety of nutritious and delicious breakfast options while being mindful of low uric acid-friendly ingredients. Enjoy your healthy meals!

5.2 Lunch Recipes

1. Grilled Chicken Salad with Avocado and Citrus Dressing

Intro: This grilled chicken salad is a refreshing and nutritious option featuring juicy grilled chicken, creamy avocado, and a zesty citrus dressing. It's perfect for a light and healthy lunch.

Total Prep Time

- 30 minutes

Ingredients

- 2 boneless, skinless chicken breasts
- 1 tablespoon olive oil
- Salt and pepper to taste
- 4 cups mixed salad greens
- 1 avocado, sliced
- 1 cup cherry tomatoes, halved
- 1/4 cup red onion, thinly sliced

Citrus Dressing

- 1/4 cup orange juice
- 2 tablespoons lemon juice
- 2 tablespoons olive oil
- 1 teaspoon honey
- Salt and pepper to taste

Instructions

1. Preheat the grill to medium-high heat.

2. Brush the chicken breasts with olive oil and season with salt and pepper.
3. Grill the chicken for 6-7 minutes on each side or until fully cooked. Let it rest for 5 minutes before slicing.
4. In a large bowl, combine the mixed salad greens, avocado, cherry tomatoes, and red onion.
5. In a small bowl, whisk together the orange juice, lemon juice, olive oil, honey, salt, and pepper to make the dressing.
6. Add the sliced chicken to the salad and drizzle with the citrus dressing.
7. Toss gently to combine and serve immediately.

Nutritional Information (per serving)

- Calories: 350
- Protein: 30g
- Carbohydrates: 20g
- Fiber: 8g
- Fat: 18g

Tips for Making it Low Uric Acid-Friendly

- Use skinless chicken breasts to reduce fat intake.
- Incorporate a variety of vegetables that are low in purines, such as mixed salad greens, avocado, and tomatoes.
- Opt for a citrus-based dressing to add flavor without high-purine ingredients.

2. Quinoa and Black Bean Salad with Lime Vinaigrette

Intro: This quinoa and black bean salad is a protein-packed and fiber-rich meal that's perfect for a quick and healthy lunch. The lime vinaigrette adds a refreshing tang to the dish.

Total Prep Time

- 25 minutes

Ingredients

- 1 cup quinoa
- 2 cups water

- 1 can black beans, drained and rinsed
- 1 cup corn kernels (fresh or frozen)
- 1 red bell pepper, diced
- 1/4 cup red onion, finely chopped
- 1/4 cup fresh cilantro, chopped

Lime Vinaigrette
- 1/4 cup fresh lime juice
- 2 tablespoons olive oil
- 1 teaspoon honey
- 1/2 teaspoon cumin
- Salt and pepper to taste

Instructions
1. Rinse the quinoa under cold water. In a medium saucepan, bring water to a boil. Add quinoa, reduce heat to low, cover, and simmer for 15 minutes or until the water is absorbed.
2. In a large bowl, combine the cooked quinoa, black beans, corn, red bell pepper, red onion, and cilantro.
3. In a small bowl, whisk together the lime juice, olive oil, honey, cumin, salt, and pepper to make the vinaigrette.
4. Pour the vinaigrette over the quinoa salad and toss to combine.
5. Serve chilled or at room temperature.

Nutritional Information (per serving)
- Calories: 280
- Protein: 10g
- Carbohydrates: 45g
- Fiber: 10g
- Fat: 8g

Tips for Making it Low Uric Acid-Friendly
- Use quinoa, which is low in purines and a good source of protein.
- Incorporate black beans and a variety of vegetables that are low in purines.

- Opt for a lime-based vinaigrette to add flavor without high-purine ingredients.

3. Roasted Vegetable Wrap with Hummus

Intro: Roasted vegetable wraps with hummus are a flavorful and nutritious lunch option. The combination of roasted vegetables and creamy hummus wrapped in a whole grain tortilla makes for a satisfying meal.

Total Prep Time

- 35 minutes

Ingredients

- 1 red bell pepper, sliced
- 1 zucchini, sliced
- 1 yellow squash, sliced
- 1 red onion, sliced
- 2 tablespoons olive oil
- Salt and pepper to taste
- 4 whole grain tortillas
- 1 cup hummus
- 2 cups mixed salad greens

Instructions

1. Preheat the oven to 425°F (220°C).
2. Place the sliced vegetables on a baking sheet and drizzle with olive oil. Season with salt and pepper.
3. Roast the vegetables for 20-25 minutes, until tender and slightly charred.
4. Spread a generous layer of hummus on each whole grain tortilla.
5. Divide the roasted vegetables and mixed salad greens among the tortillas.
6. Roll up the tortillas tightly and serve immediately.

Nutritional Information (per serving)

- Calories: 350
- Protein: 10g

- Carbohydrates: 45g
- Fiber: 8g
- Fat: 15g

Tips for Making it Low Uric Acid-Friendly

- Use whole grain tortillas to increase fiber intake.
- Incorporate a variety of roasted vegetables that are low in purines.
- Use hummus as a healthy and low-purine spread.

4. Spinach and Strawberry Salad with Poppy Seed Dressing

Intro: This spinach and strawberry salad with poppy seed dressing is a fresh and vibrant lunch option. The sweet strawberries, crunchy almonds, and tangy dressing make this salad a delightful meal.

Total Prep Time

- 15 minutes

Ingredients

- 4 cups fresh spinach
- 2 cups strawberries, sliced
- 1/4 cup red onion, thinly sliced
- 1/4 cup sliced almonds, toasted

Poppy Seed Dressing

- 1/4 cup olive oil
- 2 tablespoons apple cider vinegar
- 1 tablespoon honey
- 1 teaspoon poppy seeds
- Salt and pepper to taste

Instructions

1. In a large bowl, combine the spinach, strawberries, red onion, and toasted almonds.
2. In a small bowl, whisk together the olive oil, apple cider vinegar, honey, poppy seeds, salt, and pepper to make the dressing.
3. Pour the dressing over the salad and toss gently to combine.

4. Serve immediately.

Nutritional Information (per serving)

- Calories: 220
- Protein: 4g
- Carbohydrates: 20g
- Fiber: 5g
- Fat: 15g

Tips for Making it Low Uric Acid-Friendly

- Use fresh spinach and strawberries, which are low in purines.
- Opt for a homemade poppy seed dressing to control the ingredients and avoid high-purine additives.
- Include almonds in moderation for added crunch and nutrients.

5. Lentil and Vegetable Soup

Intro: Lentil and vegetable soup is a hearty and nutritious meal that's perfect for a cozy lunch. It's packed with protein, fiber, and a variety of vegetables, making it both delicious and healthy.

Total Prep Time

- 1 hour

Ingredients

- 1 cup lentils, rinsed
- 1 tablespoon olive oil
- 1 onion, chopped
- 2 carrots, diced
- 2 celery stalks, diced
- 2 garlic cloves, minced
- 1 can diced tomatoes
- 4 cups vegetable broth
- 1 teaspoon dried thyme
- 1 teaspoon dried oregano
- Salt and pepper to taste
- 2 cups spinach, chopped

Instructions

1. In a large pot, heat the olive oil over medium heat.
2. Add the onion, carrots, and celery, and cook until softened, about 5 minutes.
3. Add the garlic and cook for another minute.
4. Stir in the lentils, diced tomatoes, vegetable broth, thyme, oregano, salt, and pepper.
5. Bring to a boil, then reduce the heat and simmer for 30-40 minutes, until the lentils are tender.
6. Stir in the chopped spinach and cook for another 5 minutes.
7. Serve hot.

Nutritional Information (per serving)

- Calories: 250
- Protein: 12g
- Carbohydrates: 40g
- Fiber: 12g
- Fat: 5g

Tips for Making it Low Uric Acid-Friendly

- Use lentils as a low-purine source of protein and fiber.
- Incorporate a variety of low-purine vegetables.
- Opt for homemade vegetable broth to control sodium and avoid high-purine additives.

6. Greek Salad with Feta and Olives

Intro: Greek salad with feta and olives is a classic and flavorful lunch option. It combines fresh vegetables, tangy feta cheese, and briny olives for a delicious and healthy meal.

Total Prep Time

- 15 minutes

Ingredients

- 4 cups romaine lettuce, chopped
- 1 cucumber, sliced
- 1 cup cherry tomatoes, halved

- 1/2 red onion, thinly sliced
- 1/2 cup Kalamata olives
- 1/4 cup feta cheese, crumbled

Dressing

- 1/4 cup olive oil
- 2 tablespoons red wine vinegar
- 1 teaspoon dried oregano
- Salt and pepper to taste

Instructions

1. In a large bowl, combine the romaine lettuce, cucumber, cherry tomatoes, red onion, olives, and feta cheese.
2. In a small bowl, whisk together the olive oil, red wine vinegar, oregano, salt, and pepper to make the dressing.
3. Pour the dressing over the salad and toss gently to combine.
4. Serve immediately.

Nutritional Information (per serving)

- Calories: 220
- Protein: 5g
- Carbohydrates: 10g
- Fiber: 3g
- Fat: 18g

Tips for Making it Low Uric Acid-Friendly

- Use fresh vegetables that are low in purines.
- Incorporate feta cheese in moderation to add flavor without excessive dairy intake.
- Opt for a homemade dressing to control the ingredients and avoid high-purine additives.

7. Grilled Salmon with Asparagus and Lemon

Intro: Grilled salmon with asparagus and lemon is a simple yet elegant dish. This meal is packed with omega-3 fatty acids and nutrients, making it a healthy choice for lunch.

Total Prep Time

- 30 minutes

Ingredients
- 2 salmon fillets
- 1 tablespoon olive oil
- Salt and pepper to taste
- 1 bunch asparagus, trimmed
- 1 lemon, sliced

Instructions
1. Preheat the grill to medium-high heat.
2. Brush the salmon fillets with olive oil and season with salt and pepper.
3. Place the salmon fillets on the grill, skin side down, and cook for 5-6 minutes per side, or until the salmon is cooked through.
4. While the salmon is grilling, toss the asparagus with olive oil, salt, and pepper.
5. Grill the asparagus for 5-7 minutes, turning occasionally, until tender and slightly charred.
6. Serve the grilled salmon with asparagus and lemon slices on the side.

Nutritional Information (per serving)
- Calories: 350
- Protein: 30g
- Carbohydrates: 10g
- Fiber: 4g
- Fat: 20g

Tips for Making it Low Uric Acid-Friendly
- Choose fresh salmon, which is lower in purines compared to other fish.
- Incorporate asparagus, a low-purine vegetable that adds nutrients and flavor.
- Use lemon slices to enhance the flavor without adding high-purine ingredients.

8. Chickpea and Tomato Salad with Basil

Intro: Chickpea and tomato salad with basil is a light and refreshing dish. It's perfect for a quick lunch and is rich in fiber and plant-based protein.

Total Prep Time

- 15 minutes

Ingredients

- 1 can chickpeas, drained and rinsed
- 1 cup cherry tomatoes, halved
- 1/4 cup red onion, finely chopped
- 1/4 cup fresh basil, chopped
- 2 tablespoons olive oil
- 1 tablespoon balsamic vinegar
- Salt and pepper to taste

Instructions

1. In a large bowl, combine the chickpeas, cherry tomatoes, red onion, and basil.
2. In a small bowl, whisk together the olive oil, balsamic vinegar, salt, and pepper.
3. Pour the dressing over the salad and toss gently to combine.
4. Serve immediately.

Nutritional Information (per serving)

- Calories: 250
- Protein: 8g
- Carbohydrates: 30g
- Fiber: 8g
- Fat: 12g

Tips for Making it Low Uric Acid-Friendly

- Use chickpeas as a low-purine source of protein and fiber.
- Incorporate fresh tomatoes and basil, which are low in purines.
- Opt for a homemade balsamic dressing to control the ingredients.

9. Whole Grain Pasta Salad with Fresh Vegetables

Intro: Whole grain pasta salad with fresh vegetables is a nutritious and filling lunch option. It's perfect for meal prep and can be enjoyed cold or at room temperature.

Total Prep Time

- 25 minutes

Ingredients

- 2 cups whole grain pasta
- 1 cup cherry tomatoes, halved
- 1 cup cucumber, diced
- 1/2 cup red bell pepper, diced
- 1/4 cup red onion, finely chopped
- 1/4 cup black olives, sliced
- 1/4 cup feta cheese, crumbled

Dressing

- 1/4 cup olive oil
- 2 tablespoons red wine vinegar
- 1 teaspoon dried oregano
- Salt and pepper to taste

Instructions

1. Cook the pasta according to the package instructions. Drain and rinse under cold water.
2. In a large bowl, combine the cooked pasta, cherry tomatoes, cucumber, red bell pepper, red onion, black olives, and feta cheese.
3. In a small bowl, whisk together the olive oil, red wine vinegar, oregano, salt, and pepper.
4. Pour the dressing over the pasta salad and toss gently to combine.
5. Serve chilled or at room temperature.

Nutritional Information (per serving)

- Calories: 300
- Protein: 10g
- Carbohydrates: 40g

- Fiber: 8g
- Fat: 14g

Tips for Making it Low Uric Acid-Friendly
- Use whole grain pasta for added fiber and nutrients.
- Incorporate a variety of fresh vegetables that are low in purines.
- Opt for a homemade dressing to control the ingredients and avoid high-purine additives.

10. Stuffed Bell Peppers with Quinoa and Vegetables

Intro: Stuffed bell peppers with quinoa and vegetables are a colorful and nutritious lunch option. They are packed with protein, fiber, and a variety of vegetables.

Total Prep Time
- 45 minutes

Ingredients
- 4 bell peppers, tops cut off and seeds removed
- 1 cup quinoa, rinsed
- 2 cups vegetable broth
- 1 tablespoon olive oil
- 1 onion, chopped
- 2 garlic cloves, minced
- 1 zucchini, diced
- 1 cup cherry tomatoes, halved
- 1/4 cup fresh parsley, chopped
- Salt and pepper to taste

Instructions
1. Preheat the oven to 375°F (190°C).
2. In a medium saucepan, bring the vegetable broth to a boil. Add the quinoa, reduce the heat, cover, and simmer for 15 minutes or until the quinoa is cooked and the broth is absorbed.
3. In a large skillet, heat the olive oil over medium heat. Add the onion and garlic and cook until softened, about 5 minutes.

4. Add the zucchini and cherry tomatoes, and cook for another 5 minutes.
5. Stir in the cooked quinoa and parsley. Season with salt and pepper.
6. Stuff the bell peppers with the quinoa mixture and place them in a baking dish.
7. Cover the dish with foil and bake for 25-30 minutes, until the peppers are tender.
8. Serve hot.

Nutritional Information (per serving)
- Calories: 250
- Protein: 8g
- Carbohydrates: 40g
- Fiber: 10g
- Fat: 6g

Tips for Making it Low Uric Acid-Friendly
- Use quinoa as a low-purine source of protein and fiber.
- Incorporate a variety of vegetables that are low in purines.
- Opt for vegetable broth to control the ingredients and avoid high-purine additives.

11. Vegetable Stir-Fry with Brown Rice

Intro: Vegetable stir-fry with brown rice is a quick and easy lunch option that's packed with nutrients. It's a great way to incorporate a variety of vegetables into your diet.

Total Prep Time
- 30 minutes

Ingredients
- 1 cup brown rice
- 2 cups water
- 1 tablespoon olive oil
- 1 onion, chopped
- 2 garlic cloves, minced

- 1 red bell pepper, sliced
- 1 yellow bell pepper, sliced
- 1 zucchini, sliced
- 1 cup broccoli florets
- 2 tablespoons soy sauce (low sodium)
- 1 tablespoon sesame oil
- 1 teaspoon fresh ginger, grated
- 1/4 cup green onions, chopped
- 1 tablespoon sesame seeds

Instructions

1. In a medium saucepan, bring the water to a boil. Add the brown rice, reduce the heat, cover, and simmer for 20 minutes or until the rice is cooked and the water is absorbed.
2. In a large skillet, heat the olive oil over medium heat. Add the onion and garlic and cook until softened, about 5 minutes.
3. Add the red bell pepper, yellow bell pepper, zucchini, and broccoli, and cook for another 5-7 minutes, until the vegetables are tender but still crisp.
4. Stir in the soy sauce, sesame oil, and fresh ginger.
5. Serve the vegetable stir-fry over brown rice, and garnish with green onions and sesame seeds.

Nutritional Information (per serving)

- Calories: 300
- Protein: 8g
- Carbohydrates: 50g
- Fiber: 8g
- Fat: 10g

Tips for Making it Low Uric Acid-Friendly

- Use brown rice for added fiber and nutrients.
- Incorporate a variety of vegetables that are low in purines.
- Opt for low-sodium soy sauce to control sodium intake.

12. Cucumber and Avocado Sushi Rolls

Intro: Cucumber and avocado sushi rolls are a fresh and healthy lunch option. They are easy to make at home and are perfect for a light meal.

Total Prep Time

- 30 minutes

Ingredients

- 2 cups sushi rice
- 2 1/2 cups water
- 1/4 cup rice vinegar
- 2 tablespoons sugar
- 1 teaspoon salt
- 1 cucumber, julienned
- 1 avocado, sliced
- 4 sheets nori (seaweed)
- Soy sauce (for serving)
- Pickled ginger (for serving)

Instructions

1. Rinse the sushi rice under cold water until the water runs clear. In a medium saucepan, bring the rice and water to a boil. Reduce the heat to low, cover, and simmer for 20 minutes or until the rice is cooked and the water is absorbed. Let it cool slightly.
2. In a small bowl, mix the rice vinegar, sugar, and salt until the sugar is dissolved. Pour this mixture over the cooked rice and gently fold to combine.
3. Place a sheet of nori on a bamboo sushi mat. Spread an even layer of the rice over the nori, leaving a 1-inch border at the top edge.
4. Arrange the cucumber and avocado slices along the bottom edge of the rice.
5. Using the bamboo mat, roll the sushi tightly from the bottom, pressing firmly to seal. Moisten the top edge of the nori with water to seal the roll.
6. Using a sharp knife, cut the roll into 8 pieces. Repeat with the remaining ingredients.

7. Serve the sushi rolls with soy sauce and pickled ginger.

Nutritional Information (per serving)

- Calories: 200
- Protein: 4g
- Carbohydrates: 40g
- Fiber: 4g
- Fat: 6g

Tips for Making it Low Uric Acid-Friendly

- Use fresh cucumber and avocado, which are low in purines.
- Opt for low-sodium soy sauce to control sodium intake.
- Include plenty of vegetables to increase fiber and nutrients.

13. Butternut Squash Soup with Whole Grain Bread

Intro: Butternut squash soup with whole grain bread is a warm and comforting lunch option. This creamy soup is rich in vitamins and minerals, making it both delicious and healthy.

Total Prep Time

- 45 minutes

Ingredients

- 1 butternut squash, peeled, seeded, and cubed
- 1 tablespoon olive oil
- 1 onion, chopped
- 2 garlic cloves, minced
- 4 cups vegetable broth
- 1 teaspoon dried thyme
- Salt and pepper to taste
- Whole grain bread (for serving)

Instructions

1. Preheat the oven to 400°F (200°C).
2. Place the butternut squash cubes on a baking sheet and drizzle with olive oil. Roast for 25-30 minutes, until tender and lightly browned.

3. In a large pot, heat a tablespoon of olive oil over medium heat. Add the onion and garlic, and cook until softened, about 5 minutes.
4. Add the roasted butternut squash, vegetable broth, thyme, salt, and pepper. Bring to a boil, then reduce the heat and simmer for 15 minutes.
5. Use an immersion blender to puree the soup until smooth. If using a regular blender, blend the soup in batches.
6. Serve the soup hot with whole grain bread on the side.

Nutritional Information (per serving)
- Calories: 250
- Protein: 4g
- Carbohydrates: 45g
- Fiber: 8g
- Fat: 8g

Tips for Making it Low Uric Acid-Friendly
- Use butternut squash and other low-purine vegetables.
- Opt for vegetable broth to control the ingredients and avoid high-purine additives.
- Serve with whole grain bread for added fiber and nutrients.

14. Mixed Greens with Balsamic Vinaigrette and Walnuts

Intro: Mixed greens with balsamic vinaigrette and walnuts is a simple yet flavorful salad. It's perfect for a light and healthy lunch, providing a mix of textures and flavors.

Total Prep Time
- 10 minutes

Ingredients
- 4 cups mixed salad greens
- 1/2 cup cherry tomatoes, halved
- 1/4 cup red onion, thinly sliced

- 1/4 cup walnuts, toasted

Balsamic Vinaigrette

- 1/4 cup balsamic vinegar
- 2 tablespoons olive oil
- 1 teaspoon Dijon mustard
- Salt and pepper to taste

Instructions

1. In a large bowl, combine the mixed salad greens, cherry tomatoes, red onion, and toasted walnuts.
2. In a small bowl, whisk together the balsamic vinegar, olive oil, Dijon mustard, salt, and pepper to make the vinaigrette.
3. Pour the vinaigrette over the salad and toss gently to combine.
4. Serve immediately.

Nutritional Information (per serving)

- Calories: 200
- Protein: 4g
- Carbohydrates: 10g
- Fiber: 4g
- Fat: 18g

Tips for Making it Low Uric Acid-Friendly

- Use a variety of fresh salad greens and vegetables that are low in purines.
- Include walnuts in moderation for added texture and nutrients.
- Opt for a homemade balsamic vinaigrette to control the ingredients.

15. Eggplant and Zucchini Ratatouille

Intro: Eggplant and zucchini ratatouille is a hearty and flavorful vegetable stew. It's perfect for a comforting lunch and is packed with nutrients and flavor.

Total Prep Time

- 1 hour

Ingredients

- 1 eggplant, diced

- 1 zucchini, diced
- 1 red bell pepper, diced
- 1 onion, chopped
- 2 garlic cloves, minced
- 2 tablespoons olive oil
- 1 can diced tomatoes
- 1 teaspoon dried thyme
- 1 teaspoon dried oregano
- Salt and pepper to taste

Instructions

1. In a large pot, heat the olive oil over medium heat. Add the onion and garlic and cook until softened, about 5 minutes.
2. Add the eggplant, zucchini, and red bell pepper, and cook for another 10 minutes, until the vegetables are tender.
3. Stir in the diced tomatoes, thyme, oregano, salt, and pepper. Bring to a boil, then reduce the heat and simmer for 30 minutes, until the vegetables are soft and the flavors are well combined.
4. Serve hot.

Nutritional Information (per serving)

- Calories: 180
- Protein: 4g
- Carbohydrates: 20g
- Fiber: 6g
- Fat: 10g

Tips for Making it Low Uric Acid-Friendly

- Use eggplant, zucchini, and other low-purine vegetables.
- Opt for canned tomatoes without added salt or preservatives.
- Cook with olive oil to add healthy fats.

16. Turkey and Avocado Lettuce Wraps

Intro: Turkey and avocado lettuce wraps are a light and refreshing lunch option. They are easy to prepare and perfect for a quick meal on the go.

Total Prep Time

- 15 minutes

Ingredients

- 8 large lettuce leaves (such as romaine or butter lettuce)
- 8 slices deli turkey breast
- 1 avocado, sliced
- 1 tomato, sliced
- 1/4 cup red onion, thinly sliced
- Salt and pepper to taste

Instructions

1. Lay out the lettuce leaves on a flat surface.
2. Place a slice of turkey breast on each lettuce leaf.
3. Add a few slices of avocado, tomato, and red onion to each wrap.
4. Season with salt and pepper.
5. Roll up the lettuce leaves to enclose the filling.
6. Serve immediately.

Nutritional Information (per serving)

- Calories: 200
- Protein: 15g
- Carbohydrates: 10g
- Fiber: 6g
- Fat: 12g

Tips for Making it Low Uric Acid-Friendly

- Use fresh lettuce, avocado, and tomato, which are low in purines.
- Opt for deli turkey breast without added preservatives or high sodium.
- Include a variety of vegetables to increase fiber and nutrients.

17. Cauliflower Rice with Grilled Chicken and Veggies

Intro: Cauliflower rice with grilled chicken and veggies is a low-carb and nutritious lunch option. It's packed with flavor and easy to prepare.

Total Prep Time

- 30 minutes

Ingredients

- 2 chicken breasts
- 1 tablespoon olive oil
- Salt and pepper to taste
- 1 head cauliflower, grated to make cauliflower rice
- 1 red bell pepper, diced
- 1 zucchini, diced
- 1 cup broccoli florets
- 2 tablespoons soy sauce (low sodium)
- 1 teaspoon sesame oil

Instructions

1. Preheat the grill to medium-high heat.
2. Brush the chicken breasts with olive oil and season with salt and pepper.
3. Grill the chicken for 6-7 minutes on each side or until fully cooked. Let it rest for 5 minutes before slicing.
4. In a large skillet, heat the sesame oil over medium heat. Add the grated cauliflower, red bell pepper, zucchini, and broccoli, and cook for 5-7 minutes, until the vegetables are tender.
5. Stir in the soy sauce and cook for another minute.
6. Serve the cauliflower rice with sliced grilled chicken on top.

Nutritional Information (per serving)

- Calories: 350
- Protein: 30g
- Carbohydrates: 20g
- Fiber: 8g
- Fat: 16g

Tips for Making it Low Uric Acid-Friendly

- Use cauliflower rice as a low-carb and low-purine alternative to regular rice.

- Incorporate a variety of vegetables that are low in purines.
- Choose lean, skinless chicken breasts to reduce fat intake.

18. Bean and Corn Salad with Cilantro Dressing

Intro: Bean and corn salad with cilantro dressing is a vibrant and healthy lunch option. This salad is packed with protein, fiber, and fresh flavors, making it perfect for a quick meal.

Total Prep Time

- 15 minutes

Ingredients

- 1 can black beans, drained and rinsed
- 1 cup corn kernels (fresh, frozen, or canned)
- 1 red bell pepper, diced
- 1/4 cup red onion, finely chopped
- 1/4 cup fresh cilantro, chopped

Cilantro Dressing

- 1/4 cup olive oil
- 2 tablespoons lime juice
- 1 garlic clove, minced
- 1/4 teaspoon cumin
- Salt and pepper to taste

Instructions

1. In a large bowl, combine the black beans, corn, red bell pepper, red onion, and cilantro.
2. In a small bowl, whisk together the olive oil, lime juice, garlic, cumin, salt, and pepper to make the dressing.
3. Pour the dressing over the salad and toss gently to combine.
4. Serve immediately or refrigerate until ready to serve.

Nutritional Information (per serving)

- Calories: 250
- Protein: 8g

- Carbohydrates: 35g
- Fiber: 10g
- Fat: 10g

Tips for Making it Low Uric Acid-Friendly
- Use black beans and corn, which are low in purines.
- Incorporate fresh vegetables to increase fiber and nutrients.
- Opt for a homemade dressing to control the ingredients and avoid high-purine additives.

19. Tomato Basil Soup with Whole Grain Crackers

Intro: Tomato basil soup with whole grain crackers is a classic and comforting lunch option. This soup is rich in flavor and nutrients, making it a healthy choice.

Total Prep Time
- 40 minutes

Ingredients
- 1 tablespoon olive oil
- 1 onion, chopped
- 2 garlic cloves, minced
- 6 large tomatoes, chopped
- 4 cups vegetable broth
- 1/4 cup fresh basil, chopped
- Salt and pepper to taste
- Whole grain crackers (for serving)

Instructions
1. In a large pot, heat the olive oil over medium heat. Add the onion and garlic, and cook until softened, about 5 minutes.
2. Add the chopped tomatoes and cook for another 10 minutes, until the tomatoes are softened.
3. Pour in the vegetable broth and bring to a boil. Reduce the heat and simmer for 20 minutes.
4. Stir in the fresh basil and season with salt and pepper.

5. Use an immersion blender to puree the soup until smooth. If using a regular blender, blend the soup in batches.
6. Serve the soup hot with whole grain crackers on the side.

Nutritional Information (per serving)

- Calories: 200
- Protein: 4g
- Carbohydrates: 30g
- Fiber: 6g
- Fat: 8g

Tips for Making it Low Uric Acid-Friendly

- Use fresh tomatoes and basil, which are low in purines.
- Opt for vegetable broth to control the ingredients and avoid high-purine additives.
- Serve with whole grain crackers for added fiber and nutrients.

20. Roasted Beet and Goat Cheese Salad

Intro: Roasted beet and goat cheese salad is a colorful and nutritious lunch option. This salad is packed with flavor and nutrients, making it both delicious and healthy.

Total Prep Time

- 1 hour

Ingredients

- 4 medium beets, peeled and diced
- 2 tablespoons olive oil
- Salt and pepper to taste
- 4 cups mixed salad greens
- 1/4 cup goat cheese, crumbled
- 1/4 cup walnuts, toasted

Dressing

- 1/4 cup balsamic vinegar
- 2 tablespoons olive oil
- 1 teaspoon honey

- Salt and pepper to taste

Instructions

1. Preheat the oven to 400°F (200°C).
2. Place the diced beets on a baking sheet and drizzle with olive oil. Season with salt and pepper. Roast for 35-40 minutes, until tender and lightly browned.
3. In a large bowl, combine the mixed salad greens, roasted beets, goat cheese, and toasted walnuts.
4. In a small bowl, whisk together the balsamic vinegar, olive oil, honey, salt, and pepper to make the dressing.
5. Pour the dressing over the salad and toss gently to combine.
6. Serve immediately.

Nutritional Information (per serving)

- Calories: 300
- Protein: 6g
- Carbohydrates: 25g
- Fiber: 8g
- Fat: 20g

Tips for Making it Low Uric Acid-Friendly

- Use fresh beets and salad greens, which are low in purines.
- Incorporate goat cheese in moderation for added flavor without excessive dairy intake.
- Opt for a homemade balsamic dressing to control the ingredients and avoid high-purine additives

These recipes are designed to provide a variety of nutritious and delicious lunch options while being mindful of low uric acid-friendly ingredients. Enjoy your healthy meals!

5.3 Dinner Recipes

1. Baked Cod with Lemon and Dill

Intro: Baked cod with lemon and dill is a light and flavorful dinner option. This dish is quick to prepare and offers a healthy dose of omega-3 fatty acids, making it perfect for a nutritious meal.

Total Prep Time

- 30 minutes

Ingredients

- 4 cod fillets
- 2 tablespoons olive oil
- 1 lemon, sliced
- 2 tablespoons fresh dill, chopped
- Salt and pepper to taste

Instructions

1. Preheat the oven to 400°F (200°C).
2. Place the cod fillets in a baking dish and drizzle with olive oil.
3. Arrange the lemon slices on top of the fillets.
4. Sprinkle with fresh dill, salt, and pepper.
5. Bake for 20-25 minutes, until the fish is opaque and flakes easily with a fork.
6. Serve hot.

Nutritional Information (per serving)

- Calories: 200
- Protein: 30g
- Carbohydrates: 2g
- Fiber: 1g
- Fat: 8g

Tips for Making it Low Uric Acid-Friendly

- Use fresh cod, which is low in purines.
- Incorporate fresh lemon and dill to add flavor without high-purine additives.
- Serve with steamed vegetables or a side salad for added nutrients.

2. Quinoa-Stuffed Bell Peppers

Intro: Quinoa-stuffed bell peppers are a nutritious and colorful dinner option. Packed with protein and fiber, this dish is both filling and healthy.

Total Prep Time

- 50 minutes

Ingredients

- 4 large bell peppers
- 1 cup quinoa, rinsed
- 2 cups vegetable broth
- 1 can black beans, drained and rinsed
- 1 cup corn kernels (fresh, frozen, or canned)
- 1 cup diced tomatoes
- 1 teaspoon cumin
- 1 teaspoon paprika
- Salt and pepper to taste

Instructions

1. Preheat the oven to 375°F (190°C).
2. Cut the tops off the bell peppers and remove the seeds.
3. In a medium saucepan, bring the quinoa and vegetable broth to a boil. Reduce the heat, cover, and simmer for 15 minutes, until the quinoa is cooked and the liquid is absorbed.
4. In a large bowl, combine the cooked quinoa, black beans, corn, diced tomatoes, cumin, paprika, salt, and pepper.
5. Stuff the bell peppers with the quinoa mixture and place them in a baking dish.
6. Cover with foil and bake for 30 minutes. Remove the foil and bake for an additional 10 minutes.
7. Serve hot.

Nutritional Information (per serving)

- Calories: 300
- Protein: 12g
- Carbohydrates: 50g
- Fiber: 10g
- Fat: 6g

Tips for Making it Low Uric Acid-Friendly
- Use quinoa, which is low in purines and high in protein.
- Incorporate a variety of fresh vegetables for added fiber and nutrients.
- Opt for low-sodium vegetable broth to control sodium intake.

3. Grilled Tofu with Sesame and Ginger

Intro: Grilled tofu with sesame and ginger is a flavorful and protein-rich dinner option. This dish is perfect for vegetarians and those looking to reduce meat consumption.

Total Prep Time
- 30 minutes

Ingredients
- 1 block firm tofu, drained and pressed
- 2 tablespoons soy sauce (low sodium)
- 1 tablespoon sesame oil
- 1 tablespoon fresh ginger, grated
- 2 garlic cloves, minced
- 1 tablespoon sesame seeds

Instructions
1. Cut the tofu into slices and place them in a shallow dish.
2. In a small bowl, whisk together the soy sauce, sesame oil, ginger, and garlic.
3. Pour the marinade over the tofu slices and let them marinate for 15 minutes.
4. Preheat the grill to medium-high heat.
5. Grill the tofu slices for 3-4 minutes on each side, until lightly charred and heated through.
6. Sprinkle with sesame seeds before serving.

Nutritional Information (per serving)
- Calories: 200
- Protein: 16g
- Carbohydrates: 8g

- Fiber: 2g
- Fat: 14g

Tips for Making it Low Uric Acid-Friendly

- Use firm tofu, which is low in purines and high in protein.
- Incorporate fresh ginger and garlic to add flavor without high-purine additives.
- Opt for low-sodium soy sauce to control sodium intake.

4. Baked Chicken with Rosemary and Sweet Potatoes

Intro: Baked chicken with rosemary and sweet potatoes is a hearty and nutritious dinner option. This dish is easy to prepare and packed with flavor and nutrients.

Total Prep Time

- 1 hour

Ingredients

- 4 chicken breasts
- 2 tablespoons olive oil
- 2 tablespoons fresh rosemary, chopped
- 2 large sweet potatoes, peeled and diced
- Salt and pepper to taste

Instructions

1. Preheat the oven to 375°F (190°C).
2. Place the chicken breasts in a baking dish and drizzle with olive oil.
3. Sprinkle with fresh rosemary, salt, and pepper.
4. Arrange the diced sweet potatoes around the chicken.
5. Bake for 45-50 minutes, until the chicken is fully cooked and the sweet potatoes are tender.
6. Serve hot.

Nutritional Information (per serving)

- Calories: 400
- Protein: 30g
- Carbohydrates: 40g
- Fiber: 8g

- Fat: 12g

Tips for Making it Low Uric Acid-Friendly

- Use skinless chicken breasts to reduce fat intake.
- Incorporate fresh rosemary and sweet potatoes, which are low in purines.
- Serve with a side salad for added fiber and nutrients.

5. Vegetarian Chili with Kidney Beans

Intro: Vegetarian chili with kidney beans is a hearty and flavorful dinner option. Packed with protein and fiber, this dish is both filling and nutritious.

Total Prep Time

- 1 hour

Ingredients

- 1 tablespoon olive oil
- 1 onion, chopped
- 2 garlic cloves, minced
- 1 bell pepper, diced
- 1 zucchini, diced
- 1 can kidney beans, drained and rinsed
- 1 can diced tomatoes
- 2 cups vegetable broth
- 1 tablespoon chili powder
- 1 teaspoon cumin
- Salt and pepper to taste

Instructions

1. In a large pot, heat the olive oil over medium heat. Add the onion and garlic, and cook until softened, about 5 minutes.
2. Add the bell pepper and zucchini, and cook for another 5 minutes.
3. Stir in the kidney beans, diced tomatoes, vegetable broth, chili powder, cumin, salt, and pepper.
4. Bring to a boil, then reduce the heat and simmer for 30 minutes.

5. Serve hot.

Nutritional Information (per serving)
- Calories: 250
- Protein: 12g
- Carbohydrates: 40g
- Fiber: 12g
- Fat: 6g

Tips for Making it Low Uric Acid-Friendly
- Use kidney beans and fresh vegetables, which are low in purines.
- Incorporate a variety of spices for flavor without high-purine additives.
- Opt for low-sodium vegetable broth to control sodium intake.

6. Miso Soup with Tofu and Seaweed
Intro: Miso soup with tofu and seaweed is a light and nutritious dinner option. This traditional Japanese soup is rich in flavor and provides a good source of protein and minerals.

Total Prep Time
- 20 minutes

Ingredients
- 4 cups water
- 1/4 cup miso paste
- 1 block firm tofu, cubed
- 1 sheet nori (seaweed), cut into strips
- 2 green onions, sliced

Instructions
1. In a medium saucepan, bring the water to a boil.
2. Reduce the heat to low and whisk in the miso paste until dissolved.
3. Add the cubed tofu and nori strips, and cook for 5 minutes.
4. Stir in the sliced green onions and cook for another minute.
5. Serve hot.

Nutritional Information (per serving)

- Calories: 100
- Protein: 8g
- Carbohydrates: 10g
- Fiber: 2g
- Fat: 4g

Tips for Making it Low Uric Acid-Friendly

- Use firm tofu and nori, which are low in purines.
- Opt for a moderate amount of miso paste to control sodium intake.
- Incorporate fresh green onions for added flavor and nutrients.

7. Stuffed Eggplant with Couscous and Herbs

Intro: Stuffed eggplant with couscous and herbs is a flavorful and nutritious dinner option. This dish is packed with fiber and vitamins, making it both delicious and healthy.

Total Prep Time

- 1 hour

Ingredients

- 2 large eggplants
- 1 cup couscous
- 1 cup vegetable broth
- 1 tablespoon olive oil
- 1 onion, chopped
- 2 garlic cloves, minced
- 1 tomato, diced
- 1/4 cup fresh parsley, chopped
- Salt and pepper to taste

Instructions

1. Preheat the oven to 375°F (190°C).
2. Cut the eggplants in half lengthwise and scoop out the flesh, leaving a 1/2-inch shell. Chop the flesh and set aside.

3. In a medium saucepan, bring the vegetable broth to a boil. Remove from heat, stir in the couscous, cover, and let sit for 5 minutes. Fluff with a fork.
4. In a large skillet, heat the olive oil over medium heat. Add the onion and garlic, and cook until softened, about 5 minutes.
5. Add the chopped eggplant flesh and diced tomato to the skillet. Cook for another 5 minutes until the vegetables are tender.
6. Stir in the cooked couscous and chopped parsley. Season with salt and pepper to taste.
7. Spoon the couscous mixture into the eggplant shells and place them in a baking dish.
8. Cover with foil and bake for 25-30 minutes, until the eggplants are tender.
9. Serve hot.

Nutritional Information (per serving)

- Calories: 300
- Protein: 6g
- Carbohydrates: 50g
- Fiber: 12g
- Fat: 8g

Tips for Making it Low Uric Acid-Friendly

- Use fresh eggplants and herbs, which are low in purines.
- Opt for whole wheat couscous to increase fiber intake.
- Incorporate a variety of fresh vegetables for added nutrients.

8. Grilled Shrimp with Garlic and Lemon

Intro: Grilled shrimp with garlic and lemon is a simple yet flavorful dinner option. This dish is quick to prepare and packed with protein, making it perfect for a healthy meal.

Total Prep Time

- 20 minutes

Ingredients

- 1 pound large shrimp, peeled and deveined
- 2 tablespoons olive oil
- 2 garlic cloves, minced
- 1 lemon, juiced
- Salt and pepper to taste
- Fresh parsley, chopped (for garnish)

Instructions

1. In a large bowl, combine the shrimp, olive oil, garlic, lemon juice, salt, and pepper. Toss to coat the shrimp evenly.
2. Preheat the grill to medium-high heat.
3. Thread the shrimp onto skewers.
4. Grill the shrimp for 2-3 minutes on each side, until they are opaque and cooked through.
5. Garnish with fresh parsley before serving.

Nutritional Information (per serving)

- Calories: 200
- Protein: 30g
- Carbohydrates: 3g
- Fiber: 1g
- Fat: 8g

Tips for Making it Low Uric Acid-Friendly

- Use fresh shrimp, which are relatively low in purines compared to other seafood.
- Incorporate fresh lemon juice and garlic for added flavor without high-purine additives.
- Serve with a side of steamed vegetables or a light salad for added nutrients.

9. Lentil Stew with Carrots and Celery

Intro: Lentil stew with carrots and celery is a hearty and nutritious dinner option. This dish is packed with protein, fiber, and vitamins, making it both filling and healthy.

Total Prep Time

- 1 hour

Ingredients

- 1 tablespoon olive oil
- 1 onion, chopped
- 2 garlic cloves, minced
- 2 carrots, sliced
- 2 celery stalks, sliced
- 1 cup lentils, rinsed
- 4 cups vegetable broth
- 1 teaspoon thyme
- Salt and pepper to taste

Instructions

1. In a large pot, heat the olive oil over medium heat. Add the onion and garlic, and cook until softened, about 5 minutes.
2. Add the carrots and celery, and cook for another 5 minutes.
3. Stir in the lentils, vegetable broth, thyme, salt, and pepper.
4. Bring to a boil, then reduce the heat and simmer for 45 minutes, until the lentils are tender.
5. Serve hot.

Nutritional Information (per serving)

- Calories: 250
- Protein: 15g
- Carbohydrates: 40g
- Fiber: 12g
- Fat: 6g

Tips for Making it Low Uric Acid-Friendly

- Use lentils and fresh vegetables, which are low in purines.

- Incorporate fresh herbs and spices for added flavor without high-purine additives.
- Opt for low-sodium vegetable broth to control sodium intake.

10. Roasted Cauliflower Steaks with Tahini Sauce

Intro: Roasted cauliflower steaks with tahini sauce is a delicious and nutritious dinner option. This dish is easy to prepare and offers a rich, nutty flavor, making it perfect for a healthy meal.

Total Prep Time

- 40 minutes

Ingredients

- 1 large cauliflower, cut into thick slices
- 2 tablespoons olive oil
- Salt and pepper to taste
- 1/4 cup tahini
- 2 tablespoons lemon juice
- 1 garlic clove, minced
- 2 tablespoons water
- Fresh parsley, chopped (for garnish)

Instructions

1. Preheat the oven to 425°F (220°C).
2. Place the cauliflower steaks on a baking sheet and drizzle with olive oil. Season with salt and pepper.
3. Roast for 25-30 minutes, until the cauliflower is tender and golden brown.
4. In a small bowl, whisk together the tahini, lemon juice, garlic, and water until smooth.
5. Drizzle the tahini sauce over the roasted cauliflower steaks.
6. Garnish with fresh parsley before serving.

Nutritional Information (per serving)

- Calories: 200
- Protein: 6g

- Carbohydrates: 15g
- Fiber: 6g
- Fat: 14g

Tips for Making it Low Uric Acid-Friendly
- Use fresh cauliflower, which is low in purines.
- Opt for tahini made from sesame seeds, which are low in purines and high in healthy fats.
- Incorporate fresh lemon juice and garlic for added flavor without high-purine additives.

11. Zucchini Noodles with Pesto Sauce

Intro: Zucchini noodles with pesto sauce is a light and flavorful dinner option. This dish is perfect for those looking to reduce their carbohydrate intake while enjoying a delicious meal.

Total Prep Time
- 20 minutes

Ingredients
- 4 large zucchinis, spiralized
- 1/2 cup fresh basil leaves
- 1/4 cup pine nuts
- 1/4 cup grated Parmesan cheese
- 2 garlic cloves
- 1/4 cup olive oil
- Salt and pepper to taste

Instructions
1. In a food processor, combine the basil, pine nuts, Parmesan cheese, and garlic. Pulse until finely chopped.
2. With the processor running, slowly add the olive oil until the pesto is smooth. Season with salt and pepper.
3. In a large skillet, heat a small amount of olive oil over medium heat. Add the zucchini noodles and cook for 2-3 minutes, until just tender.
4. Remove from heat and toss with the pesto sauce.
5. Serve immediately.

Nutritional Information (per serving)
- Calories: 250
- Protein: 6g
- Carbohydrates: 10g
- Fiber: 4g
- Fat: 20g

Tips for Making it Low Uric Acid-Friendly
- Use fresh zucchinis, which are low in purines.
- Incorporate fresh basil and pine nuts for added flavor and healthy fats.
- Opt for a moderate amount of Parmesan cheese to control dairy intake.

12. Turkey Meatballs with Spaghetti Squash

Intro: Turkey meatballs with spaghetti squash is a healthy and delicious dinner option. This dish is a great alternative to traditional pasta and meatballs, offering a lower carbohydrate and lower fat option.

Total Prep Time
- 1 hour

Ingredients
- 1 spaghetti squash
- 1 pound ground turkey
- 1/4 cup breadcrumbs
- 1/4 cup grated Parmesan cheese
- 1 egg
- 2 garlic cloves, minced
- 1 teaspoon Italian seasoning
- Salt and pepper to taste
- 1 jar marinara sauce

Instructions
1. Preheat the oven to 375°F (190°C).

2. Cut the spaghetti squash in half lengthwise and remove the seeds. Place the halves cut-side down on a baking sheet and bake for 40-45 minutes, until tender.
3. In a large bowl, combine the ground turkey, breadcrumbs, Parmesan cheese, egg, garlic, Italian seasoning, salt, and pepper. Mix well and form into meatballs.
4. In a large skillet, heat a small amount of olive oil over medium heat. Add the meatballs and cook for 6-8 minutes, turning occasionally, until browned on all sides.
5. Add the marinara sauce to the skillet and simmer for 10-15 minutes, until the meatballs are cooked through.
6. Use a fork to scrape the flesh of the spaghetti squash into strands.
7. Serve the turkey meatballs over the spaghetti squash and top with marinara sauce.

Nutritional Information (per serving)

- Calories: 400
- Protein: 30g
- Carbohydrates: 30g
- Fiber: 6g
- Fat: 16g

Tips for Making it Low Uric Acid-Friendly

- Use ground turkey, which is lower in purines compared to red meat.
- Incorporate spaghetti squash as a low-carbohydrate alternative to pasta.
- Opt for a marinara sauce made from fresh tomatoes and herbs.

13. Sautéed Kale and White Beans

Intro: Sautéed kale and white beans is a simple and nutritious dinner option. This dish is packed with fiber, vitamins, and protein, making it both filling and healthy.

Total Prep Time

- 20 minutes

Ingredients

- 1 tablespoon olive oil
- 1 onion, chopped
- 2 garlic cloves, minced
- 1 bunch kale, stems removed and leaves chopped
- 1 can white beans (such as cannellini beans), drained and rinsed
- 1/2 cup vegetable broth
- 1/2 teaspoon red pepper flakes (optional)
- Salt and pepper to taste
- Lemon wedges (for serving)

Instructions

1. Heat olive oil in a large skillet over medium heat. Add chopped onion and cook until softened, about 3-4 minutes.
2. Add minced garlic and cook for another 1 minute until fragrant.
3. Add chopped kale to the skillet in batches, stirring until wilted.
4. Stir in drained white beans, vegetable broth, and red pepper flakes (if using). Season with salt and pepper.
5. Simmer for 5-7 minutes, stirring occasionally, until kale is tender and flavors are well combined.
6. Serve hot, garnished with a squeeze of fresh lemon juice.

Nutritional Information (per serving)

- Calories: 250
- Protein: 10g
- Carbohydrates: 40g
- Fiber: 10g
- Fat: 6g

Tips for Making it Low Uric Acid-Friendly

- Use white beans like cannellini beans, which are low in purines.
- Kale is generally low in purines and high in nutrients; however, if you have concerns, blanching kale before sautéing can reduce its purine content further.

- Limit added red pepper flakes if sensitive to spicy foods, as some people with gout find spicy foods can trigger symptoms.

14. Broiled Tilapia with Steamed Broccoli

Intro: Broiled tilapia with steamed broccoli is a light and healthy dinner option that's quick to prepare. Tilapia is a mild-flavored fish that cooks quickly under the broiler, making it ideal for a weeknight meal.

Total Prep Time

- 25 minutes

Ingredients

- 4 tilapia fillets
- 2 tablespoons olive oil
- 1 lemon, juiced
- 1 teaspoon paprika
- Salt and pepper to taste
- 1 head broccoli, cut into florets

Instructions

1. Preheat the broiler to high and line a baking sheet with foil.
2. In a small bowl, mix together olive oil, lemon juice, paprika, salt, and pepper.
3. Place tilapia fillets on the prepared baking sheet and brush with the olive oil mixture.
4. Broil tilapia for 6-8 minutes, or until fish is opaque and flakes easily with a fork.
5. While the tilapia is broiling, steam broccoli florets until tender, about 5-7 minutes.
6. Serve the broiled tilapia alongside steamed broccoli.

Nutritional Information (per serving)

- Calories: 200
- Protein: 30g
- Carbohydrates: 6g
- Fiber: 3g
- Fat: 8g

Tips for Making it Low Uric Acid-Friendly
- Tilapia is a low-purine fish choice.
- Season with herbs and lemon juice instead of high-purine sauces.
- Serve with steamed vegetables like broccoli for added nutrients and fiber.

15. Butternut Squash Risotto
Intro: Butternut squash risotto is a creamy and comforting dinner option that's perfect for cooler evenings. This dish combines the natural sweetness of butternut squash with creamy Arborio rice for a satisfying meal.
Total Prep Time
- 45 minutes

Ingredients
- 1 small butternut squash, peeled, seeded, and diced
- 2 tablespoons olive oil
- 1 onion, finely chopped
- 2 garlic cloves, minced
- 1 cup Arborio rice
- 1/2 cup white wine (optional)
- 4 cups vegetable broth, heated
- 1/2 cup grated Parmesan cheese
- Salt and pepper to taste
- Fresh sage leaves, chopped (for garnish)

Instructions
1. Preheat the oven to 400°F (200°C).
2. Toss diced butternut squash with 1 tablespoon olive oil and spread evenly on a baking sheet. Roast for 20-25 minutes, or until squash is tender and lightly caramelized.
3. In a large skillet, heat remaining olive oil over medium heat. Add chopped onion and cook until softened, about 5 minutes.
4. Add minced garlic and Arborio rice to the skillet. Stir to coat the rice with oil.

5. If using, pour in white wine and cook until wine is absorbed, stirring constantly.
6. Gradually add hot vegetable broth, one ladleful at a time, stirring frequently and allowing each addition to be absorbed before adding more.
7. When rice is creamy and tender (about 20-25 minutes), stir in roasted butternut squash and Parmesan cheese.
8. Season with salt and pepper to taste.
9. Serve hot, garnished with chopped sage leaves.

Nutritional Information (per serving)

- Calories: 400
- Protein: 10g
- Carbohydrates: 60g
- Fiber: 6g
- Fat: 12g

Tips for Making it Low Uric Acid-Friendly

- Use Arborio rice, which is lower in purines compared to other types of rice.
- Butternut squash is generally low in purines and adds natural sweetness.
- Limit the amount of Parmesan cheese if watching dairy intake.

16. Chickpea and Spinach Curry

Intro: Chickpea and spinach curry is a flavorful and protein-rich dinner option. This vegetarian dish is packed with spices and nutrients, making it both satisfying and nutritious.

Total Prep Time

- 30 minutes

Ingredients

- 1 tablespoon olive oil
- 1 onion, finely chopped
- 2 garlic cloves, minced

- 1 tablespoon fresh ginger, grated
- 1 tablespoon curry powder
- 1 teaspoon ground cumin
- 1/2 teaspoon ground turmeric
- 1/4 teaspoon cayenne pepper (optional)
- 1 can chickpeas, drained and rinsed
- 1 can diced tomatoes
- 1 cup coconut milk
- 4 cups fresh spinach leaves
- Salt and pepper to taste

Instructions

1. In a large skillet, heat olive oil over medium heat. Add chopped onion and cook until softened, about 5 minutes.
2. Add minced garlic, grated ginger, curry powder, ground cumin, ground turmeric, and cayenne pepper (if using). Cook for 1 minute until fragrant.
3. Stir in drained chickpeas, diced tomatoes (with juice), and coconut milk. Bring to a simmer.
4. Add fresh spinach leaves and cook until wilted, about 3-5 minutes.
5. Season with salt and pepper to taste.
6. Serve hot, optionally with rice or naan bread.

Nutritional Information (per serving)

- Calories: 300
- Protein: 10g
- Carbohydrates: 30g
- Fiber: 8g
- Fat: 16g

Tips for Making it Low Uric Acid-Friendly

- Use chickpeas, which are low in purines and high in protein.
- Incorporate fresh spinach for added vitamins and minerals.
- Limit added cayenne pepper if sensitive to spicy foods.

17. Grilled Vegetable Skewers with Quinoa

Intro: Grilled vegetable skewers with quinoa are a colorful and nutritious dinner option. This dish combines marinated vegetables with protein-rich quinoa for a satisfying and flavorful meal.

Total Prep Time

- 40 minutes

Ingredients

- 1 zucchini, sliced
- 1 yellow bell pepper, cut into chunks
- 1 red bell pepper, cut into chunks
- 1 red onion, cut into chunks
- 8-10 cherry tomatoes
- 1 cup quinoa, rinsed
- 2 cups vegetable broth
- 2 tablespoons olive oil
- 2 tablespoons balsamic vinegar
- 2 garlic cloves, minced
- Salt and pepper to taste
- Fresh parsley, chopped (for garnish)

Instructions

1. In a large bowl, combine sliced zucchini, yellow bell pepper chunks, red bell pepper chunks, red onion chunks, and cherry tomatoes.
2. In a small bowl, whisk together olive oil, balsamic vinegar, minced garlic, salt, and pepper.
3. Pour the marinade over the vegetables and toss to coat. Let marinate for 15-20 minutes.
4. Meanwhile, in a medium saucepan, bring vegetable broth to a boil. Add quinoa, reduce heat to low, cover, and simmer for 15 minutes or until quinoa is cooked and liquid is absorbed.
5. Preheat the grill to medium-high heat. Thread marinated vegetables onto skewers.

6. Grill skewers for 10-12 minutes, turning occasionally, until vegetables are tender and lightly charred.
7. Fluff cooked quinoa with a fork and serve with grilled vegetable skewers.
8. Garnish with fresh parsley before serving.

Nutritional Information (per serving)

- Calories: 300
- Protein: 10g
- Carbohydrates: 50g
- Fiber: 8g
- Fat: 8g

Tips for Making it Low Uric Acid-Friendly

- Choose vegetables like zucchini, bell peppers, and tomatoes which are low in purines.
- Use quinoa as a protein source instead of high-purine meats.
- Limit added salt in the marinade to control sodium intake.

18. Roasted Brussels Sprouts and Chicken Thighs

Intro: Roasted Brussels sprouts and chicken thighs is a hearty and nutritious dinner option. This dish combines tender chicken thighs with roasted Brussels sprouts for a flavorful and satisfying meal.

Total Prep Time

- 45 minutes

Ingredients

- 4 chicken thighs, bone-in and skin-on
- 1 pound Brussels sprouts, trimmed and halved
- 2 tablespoons olive oil
- 2 garlic cloves, minced
- 1 teaspoon smoked paprika
- Salt and pepper to taste
- Fresh thyme leaves, for garnish

Instructions

1. Preheat the oven to 400°F (200°C).
2. In a large bowl, toss Brussels sprouts with olive oil, minced garlic, smoked paprika, salt, and pepper.
3. Spread Brussels sprouts evenly on a baking sheet.
4. Place chicken thighs on the baking sheet with Brussels sprouts, skin-side up. Brush chicken thighs with a little olive oil and season with salt and pepper.
5. Roast in the preheated oven for 30-35 minutes, or until chicken thighs are cooked through and Brussels sprouts are caramelized and tender.
6. Remove from oven and let rest for 5 minutes before serving.
7. Garnish with fresh thyme leaves before serving.

Nutritional Information (per serving)

- Calories: 400
- Protein: 30g
- Carbohydrates: 10g
- Fiber: 4g
- Fat: 25g

Tips for Making it Low Uric Acid-Friendly

- Use chicken thighs, which are lower in purines compared to red meats.
- Roasted Brussels sprouts are generally low in purines and rich in nutrients.
- Season with herbs and spices instead of high-purine sauces.

19. Herbed Lentil and Brown Rice Pilaf

Intro: Herbed lentil and brown rice pilaf is a wholesome and nutritious dish that combines protein-packed lentils with fiber-rich brown rice. This pilaf is flavored with herbs and spices for a delicious and satisfying meal.

Total Prep Time

- 1 hour

Ingredients

- 1 cup brown rice
- 1/2 cup green or brown lentils, rinsed
- 2 cups vegetable broth
- 2 tablespoons olive oil
- 1 onion, finely chopped
- 2 garlic cloves, minced
- 1 teaspoon dried thyme
- 1 teaspoon dried rosemary
- Salt and pepper to taste
- Fresh parsley, chopped (for garnish)

Instructions

1. In a medium saucepan, heat olive oil over medium heat. Add chopped onion and cook until softened, about 5 minutes.
2. Add minced garlic, dried thyme, and dried rosemary. Cook for 1 minute until fragrant.
3. Add brown rice and lentils to the saucepan. Stir to coat with oil and herbs.
4. Pour in vegetable broth and bring to a boil. Reduce heat to low, cover, and simmer for 40-45 minutes, or until rice and lentils are tender and liquid is absorbed.
5. Remove from heat and let pilaf stand covered for 5 minutes.
6. Fluff pilaf with a fork and season with salt and pepper to taste.
7. Garnish with fresh parsley before serving.

Nutritional Information (per serving)

- Calories: 300
- Protein: 10g
- Carbohydrates: 50g
- Fiber: 8g
- Fat: 8g

Tips for Making it Low Uric Acid-Friendly

- Use brown rice and lentils, which are lower in purines compared to white rice and some other legumes.

- Season with dried herbs for flavor instead of high-purine sauces or additives.
- Limit added salt to control sodium intake.

20. Sweet and Sour Tempeh with Pineapple

Intro: Sweet and sour tempeh with pineapple is a tangy and flavorful dish that's both vegetarian and protein-rich. This dish combines tempeh, a fermented soybean product, with sweet pineapple and a savory sauce for a delicious meal.

Total Prep Time

- 30 minutes

Ingredients

- 1 package (8 oz) tempeh, cut into cubes
- 1 cup pineapple chunks (fresh or canned)
- 1 red bell pepper, cut into chunks
- 1 onion, cut into chunks
- 2 tablespoons soy sauce (or tamari for gluten-free)
- 2 tablespoons rice vinegar
- 2 tablespoons ketchup
- 1 tablespoon brown sugar
- 1 tablespoon cornstarch
- 1/2 cup water
- 2 tablespoons vegetable oil
- Cooked rice (for serving)

Instructions

1. In a small bowl, whisk together soy sauce, rice vinegar, ketchup, brown sugar, cornstarch, and water to make the sauce. Set aside.
2. In a large skillet or wok, heat vegetable oil over medium-high heat. Add cubed tempeh and cook until golden brown on all sides, about 5 minutes. Remove tempeh from skillet and set aside.
3. In the same skillet, add pineapple chunks, red bell pepper chunks, and onion chunks. Stir-fry for 3-4 minutes until vegetables are slightly tender.

4. Return cooked tempeh to the skillet with the vegetables.
5. Pour the sauce over the tempeh and vegetables. Stir well to coat and bring to a simmer.
6. Cook for 2-3 minutes until the sauce thickens and coats the tempeh and vegetables.
7. Serve hot over cooked rice.

Nutritional Information (per serving)

- Calories: 350
- Protein: 15g
- Carbohydrates: 45g
- Fiber: 6g
- Fat: 14g

Tips for Making it Low Uric Acid-Friendly

- Tempeh is made from fermented soybeans and is generally lower in purines compared to other protein sources like meat.
- Use fresh pineapple chunks, which are low in purines and add natural sweetness.
- Opt for low-sodium soy sauce to control sodium intake.

These recipes are designed to provide a variety of nutritious and delicious Dinner options while being mindful of low uric acid-friendly ingredients. Enjoy your healthy meals!

5.4 Snack Recipes

1. Apple Slices with Almond Butter

Intro: Apple slices with almond butter make for a delicious and nutritious snack that combines the sweetness of apples with the rich, nutty flavor of almond butter.

Total Prep Time

- 5 minutes

Ingredients

- 1 apple, sliced
- 2 tablespoons almond butter

Instructions

1. Slice the apple into thin wedges.
2. Spread almond butter on each apple slice.
3. Serve immediately.

Nutritional Information (per serving)

- Calories: 180
- Protein: 4g
- Carbohydrates: 20g
- Fiber: 5g
- Fat: 10g

Tips for Making it Low Uric Acid-Friendly

- Apples are low in purines and high in fiber.
- Choose almond butter without added sugars or salt to keep it healthy.

2. **Hummus with Carrot and Cucumber Sticks**

Intro: Hummus with carrot and cucumber sticks is a crunchy and satisfying snack that's packed with vitamins and fiber, complemented by the creamy texture of hummus.

Total Prep Time

- 10 minutes

Ingredients

- 1 cup hummus
- 2 carrots, cut into sticks
- 1 cucumber, cut into sticks

Instructions

1. Arrange carrot and cucumber sticks on a plate.
2. Serve with hummus for dipping.

Nutritional Information (per serving)

- Calories: 200
- Protein: 8g
- Carbohydrates: 20g
- Fiber: 8g
- Fat: 10g

Tips for Making it Low Uric Acid-Friendly

- Carrots and cucumbers are low-purine vegetables.
- Opt for homemade or low-sodium hummus to control salt intake.

3. Mixed Nuts and Dried Fruit Trail Mix

Intro: Mixed nuts and dried fruit trail mix is a portable snack that provides a mix of protein, healthy fats, and natural sweetness from dried fruits.

Total Prep Time

- 5 minutes

Ingredients

- 1 cup mixed nuts (almonds, walnuts, cashews)
- 1/2 cup dried fruits (raisins, cranberries, apricots)

Instructions

1. Combine mixed nuts and dried fruits in a bowl.
2. Mix well.
3. Portion into individual servings for easy snacking.

Nutritional Information (per serving)

- Calories: 250
- Protein: 8g
- Carbohydrates: 25g
- Fiber: 5g
- Fat: 15g

Tips for Making it Low Uric Acid-Friendly

- Choose nuts like almonds and cashews, which are lower in purines.
- Opt for dried fruits without added sugars.

4. Baked Kale Chips

Intro: Baked kale chips are a crunchy and flavorful snack that's easy to make and packed with vitamins and minerals from kale.

Total Prep Time

- 20 minutes

Ingredients

- 1 bunch kale, stems removed and torn into pieces
- 1 tablespoon olive oil
- Salt and pepper to taste

Instructions

1. Preheat the oven to 325°F (160°C).
2. Toss kale pieces with olive oil, salt, and pepper in a bowl until evenly coated.
3. Spread kale in a single layer on a baking sheet.
4. Bake for 12-15 minutes, or until kale is crispy and edges are lightly browned.
5. Let cool before serving.

Nutritional Information (per serving)

- Calories: 150
- Protein: 5g
- Carbohydrates: 10g
- Fiber: 3g
- Fat: 10g

Tips for Making it Low Uric Acid-Friendly

- Kale is generally low in purines and high in nutrients.
- Avoid excessive salt when seasoning to control sodium intake.

5. Greek Yogurt with Honey and Blueberries

Intro: Greek yogurt with honey and blueberries is a creamy and satisfying snack that provides protein, probiotics, and antioxidants from blueberries.

Total Prep Time

- 5 minutes

Ingredients

- 1 cup Greek yogurt
- 1 tablespoon honey
- 1/2 cup fresh blueberries

Instructions

1. Spoon Greek yogurt into a bowl.
2. Drizzle honey over the yogurt.
3. Top with fresh blueberries.
4. Serve immediately.

Nutritional Information (per serving)

- Calories: 200
- Protein: 20g
- Carbohydrates: 30g
- Fiber: 2g
- Fat: 0g

Tips for Making it Low Uric Acid-Friendly

- Greek yogurt is a good source of protein with low purine content.
- Use fresh blueberries, which are low in purines and high in antioxidants.

6. Rice Cakes with Avocado and Tomato

Intro: Rice cakes with avocado and tomato are a light and crunchy snack that combines the creaminess of avocado with the freshness of tomatoes.

Total Prep Time

- 10 minutes

Ingredients

- 2 rice cakes
- 1 ripe avocado, mashed
- 1 tomato, sliced
- Salt and pepper to taste

Instructions

1. Spread mashed avocado evenly on each rice cake.
2. Top with sliced tomatoes.

3. Season with salt and pepper.
4. Serve immediately.

Nutritional Information (per serving)

- Calories: 180
- Protein: 3g
- Carbohydrates: 20g
- Fiber: 5g
- Fat: 10g

Tips for Making it Low Uric Acid-Friendly

- Rice cakes are low in purines and provide a crunchy base.
- Avocado and tomatoes are low-purine choices for toppings.

7. Roasted Chickpeas with Spices

Intro: Roasted chickpeas with spices are a crunchy and protein-packed snack that's seasoned with flavorful spices for a satisfying munch.

Total Prep Time

- 45 minutes (including baking time)

Ingredients

- 1 can (15 oz) chickpeas, drained and rinsed
- 1 tablespoon olive oil
- 1 teaspoon paprika
- 1/2 teaspoon cumin
- 1/2 teaspoon garlic powder
- Salt to taste

Instructions

- Preheat the oven to 400°F (200°C).
- Pat dry chickpeas with a paper towel to remove excess moisture.
- In a bowl, toss chickpeas with olive oil, paprika, cumin, garlic powder, and salt until evenly coated.
- Spread chickpeas in a single layer on a baking sheet.
- Bake for 30-35 minutes, shaking the pan halfway through, until chickpeas are crispy.

- Let cool before serving.

Nutritional Information (per serving)

- Calories: 200
- Protein: 8g
- Carbohydrates: 30g
- Fiber: 8g
- Fat: 5g

Tips for Making it Low Uric Acid-Friendly

- Chickpeas are low in purines and high in fiber and protein.
- Use minimal salt or opt for salt-free seasoning blends.

8. Sliced Bell Peppers with Hummus

Intro: Sliced bell peppers with hummus are a refreshing and crunchy snack that pairs the natural sweetness of bell peppers with the creamy texture of hummus.

Total Prep Time

- 10 minutes

Ingredients

- 2 bell peppers (any color), sliced
- 1 cup hummus

Instructions

1. Arrange bell pepper slices on a plate.
2. Serve with hummus for dipping.

Nutritional Information (per serving)

- Calories: 150
- Protein: 6g
- Carbohydrates: 20g
- Fiber: 8g
- Fat: 7g

Tips for Making it Low Uric Acid-Friendly

- Bell peppers are low in purines and high in vitamin C.
- Choose homemade or low-sodium hummus.

9. Celery Sticks with Peanut Butter

Intro: Celery sticks with peanut butter are a classic snack that combines the crunchiness of celery with the creamy richness of peanut butter.

Total Prep Time

- 5 minutes

Ingredients

- 4 celery stalks, cut into sticks
- 4 tablespoons natural peanut butter

Instructions

1. Spread peanut butter inside each celery stick.
2. Serve immediately.

Nutritional Information (per serving)

- Calories: 200
- Protein: 8g
- Carbohydrates: 10g
- Fiber: 4g
- Fat: 15g

Tips for Making it Low Uric Acid-Friendly

- Choose natural peanut butter without added sugars or salt.
- Celery is low in purines and adds crunch and fiber to the snack.

10. Fresh Fruit Salad with Mint

Intro: Fresh fruit salad with mint is a vibrant and refreshing dish that combines a variety of seasonal fruits with a hint of mint. This simple yet delightful recipe is perfect for a light snack, a healthy dessert, or a refreshing breakfast option. It is not only delicious but also packed with vitamins, minerals, and antioxidants.

Total Prep Time

- 15 minutes

Ingredients

- 1 cup strawberries, hulled and sliced
- 1 cup blueberries

- 1 cup pineapple, diced
- 1 cup mango, diced
- 1 cup kiwi, peeled and sliced
- 1 cup grapes, halved
- Juice of 1 lime
- 2 tablespoons honey or agave syrup (optional)
- 2 tablespoons fresh mint leaves, finely chopped

Instructions

1. Wash all the fruits thoroughly. Hull and slice the strawberries, dice the pineapple and mango, peel and slice the kiwi, and halve the grapes.
2. In a large bowl, combine all the prepared fruits.
3. Drizzle the lime juice over the fruit mixture. If desired, add honey or agave syrup for extra sweetness.
4. Sprinkle the finely chopped mint leaves over the fruit salad.
5. Gently toss the fruit salad to mix all the ingredients evenly. Serve immediately for the freshest taste.

Nutritional Information (per serving)

- Calories: 120
- Protein: 1g
- Carbohydrates: 30g
- Fiber: 4g
- Fat: 0g

Tips for Making it Low Uric Acid-Friendly

- All the fruits in this recipe are low in purines, making them suitable for a low uric acid diet.
- The high water content in fruits like pineapple and strawberries helps with hydration, which is beneficial for managing uric acid levels.
- Use honey or agave syrup sparingly as natural sweeteners. They are lower in purines compared to processed sugars.
- Mint is not only refreshing but also aids digestion and can help reduce inflammation.

11. Whole Grain Crackers with Cheese

Intro: Whole grain crackers with cheese make for a satisfying and balanced snack that combines the crunchiness of crackers with the creamy goodness of cheese.

Total Prep Time

- 5 minutes

Ingredients

- 6 whole grain crackers
- 2 ounces cheese of your choice (cheddar, Swiss, or goat cheese)

Instructions

1. Place whole grain crackers on a plate.
2. Top each cracker with a slice of cheese.
3. Serve immediately.

Nutritional Information (per serving)

- Calories: 200
- Protein: 10g
- Carbohydrates: 15g
- Fiber: 3g
- Fat: 12g

Tips for Making it Low Uric Acid-Friendly

- Opt for low-fat cheese options to reduce saturated fat intake.
- Whole grain crackers are a better choice than white flour crackers for managing uric acid levels.

12. Edamame with Sea Salt

Intro: Edamame with sea salt is a simple and nutritious snack that provides plant-based protein and fiber, perfect for a quick and healthy munch.

Total Prep Time

- 10 minutes

Ingredients

- 1 cup edamame (fresh or frozen)
- Sea salt to taste

Instructions

1. If using frozen edamame, steam or boil according to package instructions until tender.
2. Drain and sprinkle with sea salt.
3. Serve warm or chilled.

Nutritional Information (per serving)

- Calories: 120
- Protein: 11g
- Carbohydrates: 10g
- Fiber: 5g
- Fat: 4g

Tips for Making it Low Uric Acid-Friendly

- Edamame is low in purines and high in protein.
- Use sea salt sparingly to control sodium intake.

13. Homemade Popcorn with Nutritional Yeast

Intro: Homemade popcorn with nutritional yeast is a savory and crunchy snack that's rich in flavor and nutrients, making it a healthier alternative to buttered popcorn.

Total Prep Time

- 10 minutes

Ingredients

- 1/2 cup popcorn kernels
- 2 tablespoons olive oil
- 2 tablespoons nutritional yeast
- Salt to taste

Instructions

1. Heat olive oil in a large pot over medium heat.
2. Add popcorn kernels and cover with a lid.
3. Shake the pot occasionally until popping slows down.
4. Remove from heat and transfer popcorn to a large bowl.
5. Drizzle olive oil over popcorn and toss with nutritional yeast and salt.

6. Serve immediately.

Nutritional Information (per serving)

- Calories: 150
- Protein: 4g
- Carbohydrates: 20g
- Fiber: 4g
- Fat: 7g

Tips for Making it Low Uric Acid-Friendly

- Air-popped popcorn is lower in fat and calories compared to microwave popcorn.
- Nutritional yeast adds a cheesy flavor without dairy and is low in purines.

14. Cottage Cheese with Pineapple

Intro: Cottage cheese with pineapple is a creamy and refreshing snack that combines the protein-packed goodness of cottage cheese with the natural sweetness of pineapple.

Total Prep Time

- 5 minutes

Ingredients

- 1 cup cottage cheese
- 1 cup pineapple chunks (fresh or canned)

Instructions

1. Spoon cottage cheese into a bowl.
2. Top with pineapple chunks.
3. Serve immediately.

Nutritional Information (per serving)

- Calories: 180
- Protein: 20g
- Carbohydrates: 20g
- Fiber: 2g
- Fat: 2g

Tips for Making it Low Uric Acid-Friendly

- Cottage cheese is low in purines and high in protein.
- Choose fresh pineapple or canned pineapple in natural juice to avoid added sugars.

15. Baked Sweet Potato Fries

Intro: Baked sweet potato fries are a healthier alternative to traditional fries, offering a crispy texture and sweet flavor while being rich in vitamins and fiber.

Total Prep Time

- 30 minutes

Ingredients

- 2 large sweet potatoes, peeled and cut into fries
- 2 tablespoons olive oil
- 1 teaspoon paprika
- Salt and pepper to taste

Instructions

1. Preheat the oven to 425°F (220°C).
2. In a large bowl, toss sweet potato fries with olive oil, paprika, salt, and pepper until evenly coated.
3. Spread fries in a single layer on a baking sheet.
4. Bake for 20-25 minutes, flipping halfway through, until fries are crispy and golden brown.
5. Remove from oven and let cool slightly before serving.

Nutritional Information (per serving)

- Calories: 200
- Protein: 3g
- Carbohydrates: 30g
- Fiber: 5g
- Fat: 8g

Tips for Making it Low Uric Acid-Friendly

- Sweet potatoes are low in purines and packed with nutrients.
- Bake instead of frying to reduce oil content and make it healthier.

These snack recipes provide a variety of flavors and textures while being mindful of maintaining a low uric acid diet. Enjoy these nutritious snacks as part of your balanced eating plan!

5.5 Dessert Recipes

1. Chia Seed Pudding with Coconut Milk

Intro: Chia seed pudding with coconut milk is a creamy and nutritious dessert that's packed with omega-3 fatty acids and fiber from chia seeds, combined with the rich flavor of coconut milk.

Total Prep Time

- 5 minutes (plus chilling time)

Ingredients

- 1/4 cup chia seeds
- 1 cup coconut milk
- 1 tablespoon honey or maple syrup (optional)
- Fresh berries for topping

Instructions

In a bowl, mix chia seeds and coconut milk.

Add honey or maple syrup if desired for sweetness.

1. Stir well to combine, ensuring no clumps of chia seeds remain.
2. Cover and refrigerate for at least 2 hours or overnight until it reaches a pudding-like consistency.
3. Serve chilled, topped with fresh berries.

Nutritional Information (per serving)

- Calories: 250
- Protein: 5g
- Carbohydrates: 20g
- Fiber: 10g
- Fat: 15g

Tips for Making it Low Uric Acid-Friendly

- Chia seeds are low in purines and high in fiber.

- Use unsweetened coconut milk to avoid added sugars.

2. Mixed Berry Parfait with Greek Yogurt

Intro: Mixed berry parfait with Greek yogurt is a refreshing and satisfying dessert that layers creamy Greek yogurt with sweet, antioxidant-rich berries and crunchy granola.

Total Prep Time

- 10 minutes

Ingredients

- 1 cup mixed berries (strawberries, blueberries, raspberries)
- 1 cup Greek yogurt
- 1/2 cup granola
- Honey or maple syrup (optional, for sweetness)

Instructions

1. In a serving glass or bowl, layer Greek yogurt, mixed berries, and granola.
2. Repeat layers until ingredients are used up.
3. Drizzle honey or maple syrup over the top if desired.
4. Serve immediately.

Nutritional Information (per serving)

- Calories: 300
- Protein: 20g
- Carbohydrates: 40g
- Fiber: 5g
- Fat: 8g

Tips for Making it Low Uric Acid-Friendly

- Greek yogurt is low in purines and high in protein.
- Choose fresh or frozen berries without added sugars.

3. Baked Apples with Cinnamon and Raisins

Intro: Baked apples with cinnamon and raisins are a warm and comforting dessert that highlights the natural sweetness of apples, enhanced with cinnamon spice and plump raisins.

Total Prep Time

- 30 minutes

Ingredients

- 4 apples (such as Granny Smith or Honeycrisp), cored
- 1/4 cup raisins
- 1 teaspoon ground cinnamon
- 2 tablespoons honey or maple syrup (optional)
- 1/4 cup water

Instructions

1. Preheat the oven to 375°F (190°C).
2. In a small bowl, mix raisins with cinnamon.
3. Stuff each cored apple with the raisin mixture.
4. Place stuffed apples in a baking dish.
5. Drizzle honey or maple syrup over the apples if desired.
6. Pour water into the baking dish around the apples.
7. Bake for 25-30 minutes, until apples are tender.
8. Serve warm.

Nutritional Information (per serving)

- Calories: 150
- Protein: 1g
- Carbohydrates: 40g
- Fiber: 5g
- Fat: 0g

Tips for Making it Low Uric Acid-Friendly

- Apples are low in purines and high in fiber.
- Use cinnamon and honey/maple syrup sparingly for sweetness.

4. Mango Sorbet

Intro: Mango sorbet is a refreshing and tropical dessert that's naturally sweet and dairy-free, perfect for cooling down on a hot day.

Total Prep Time

- 5 minutes (plus freezing time)

Ingredients

- 2 ripe mangoes, peeled and diced
- 1/4 cup water
- 2 tablespoons honey or agave syrup (optional)

Instructions

- Place diced mangoes in a blender or food processor.
- Add water and honey/agave syrup if using.
- Blend until smooth.
- Pour mixture into a shallow dish and freeze for 4-6 hours, stirring occasionally, until firm.
- Scoop sorbet into bowls and serve.

Nutritional Information (per serving)

- Calories: 150
- Protein: 1g
- Carbohydrates: 40g
- Fiber: 3g
- Fat: 0g

Tips for Making it Low Uric Acid-Friendly

- Mangoes are low in purines and provide natural sweetness.
- Skip added sweeteners if mangoes are ripe and sweet enough.

5. Dark Chocolate and Walnut Bark

Intro: Dark chocolate and walnut bark is a decadent yet wholesome dessert that combines the antioxidant-rich goodness of dark chocolate with the crunch of walnuts.

Total Prep Time

- 15 minutes (plus cooling time)

Ingredients

- 8 ounces dark chocolate (70% cocoa or higher), chopped
- 1/2 cup walnuts, chopped

Instructions

1. Line a baking sheet with parchment paper.
2. Melt dark chocolate in a heatproof bowl set over a pot of simmering water (double boiler method), stirring until smooth.
3. Pour melted chocolate onto the prepared baking sheet, spreading it into a thin layer.
4. Sprinkle chopped walnuts evenly over the chocolate.
5. Place in the refrigerator for 1-2 hours, or until firm.
6. Once set, break or cut into pieces.
7. Serve chilled or at room temperature.

Nutritional Information (per serving)

- Calories: 200
- Protein: 3g
- Carbohydrates: 15g
- Fiber: 3g
- Fat: 15g

Tips for Making it Low Uric Acid-Friendly

- Dark chocolate is lower in purines compared to milk chocolate.
- Walnuts are moderate in purines but rich in omega-3 fatty acids.

6. Banana and Almond Butter Ice Cream

Intro: Banana and almond butter ice cream is a creamy and dairy-free dessert that's naturally sweetened with bananas and enriched with the nutty flavor of almond butter.

Total Prep Time

- 5 minutes (plus freezing time)

Ingredients

- 4 ripe bananas, sliced and frozen
- 1/4 cup almond butter
- 1 teaspoon vanilla extract (optional)

Instructions

1. Place frozen banana slices, almond butter, and vanilla extract (if using) in a blender or food processor.
2. Blend until smooth and creamy, scraping down the sides as needed.
3. Transfer mixture to a freezer-safe container.
4. Freeze for at least 2-3 hours until firm.
5. Scoop ice cream into bowls and serve.

Nutritional Information (per serving)

- Calories: 250
- Protein: 5g
- Carbohydrates: 35g
- Fiber: 5g
- Fat: 12g

Tips for Making it Low Uric Acid-Friendly

- Bananas are low in purines and provide natural sweetness.
- Use natural almond butter without added sugars or salt.

7. Coconut Rice Pudding

Intro: Coconut rice pudding is a creamy and comforting dessert made with coconut milk and aromatic jasmine rice, infused with vanilla and a hint of sweetness.

Total Prep Time

- 45 minutes

Ingredients

- 1 cup jasmine rice
- 1 can (13.5 oz) coconut milk
- 2 cups water
- 1/4 cup sugar or sweetener of choice
- 1 teaspoon vanilla extract
- Ground cinnamon for garnish (optional)

Instructions

1. Rinse jasmine rice under cold water until water runs clear.
2. In a medium saucepan, combine rinsed rice, coconut milk, water, sugar, and vanilla extract.

3. Bring mixture to a boil over medium-high heat.
4. Reduce heat to low, cover, and simmer for 30-35 minutes, stirring occasionally, until rice is tender and liquid is absorbed.
5. Remove from heat and let pudding cool slightly.
6. Serve warm or chilled, sprinkled with ground cinnamon if desired.

Nutritional Information (per serving)
- Calories: 300
- Protein: 4g
- Carbohydrates: 50g
- Fiber: 1g
- Fat: 10g

Tips for Making it Low Uric Acid-Friendly
- Use low-fat coconut milk to reduce saturated fat content.
- Adjust sweetness level to taste with less sugar or natural sweeteners.

8. Fresh Fruit Tart with Almond Crust

Intro: Fresh fruit tart with almond crust is a beautiful and fruity dessert that features a nutty almond crust filled with creamy yogurt or custard and topped with seasonal fresh fruits.

Total Prep Time
- 1 hour (including chilling time)

Ingredients

For the Almond Crust:
- 1 cup almond flour
- 1/4 cup coconut oil, melted
- 2 tablespoons honey or maple syrup
- 1/2 teaspoon vanilla extract

For the Filling and Topping:
- 1 cup Greek yogurt or custard
- Assorted fresh fruits (berries, kiwi, mango, etc.)
- 2 tablespoons apricot preserves or honey (for glaze)

Instructions

For the Almond Crust:
1. Preheat the oven to 350°F (175°C). Grease a tart pan with removable bottom.
2. In a bowl, mix almond flour, melted coconut oil, honey or maple syrup, and vanilla extract until well combined.
3. Press the mixture evenly into the greased tart pan, covering the bottom and sides.
4. Bake the crust for 10-12 minutes, until lightly golden brown.
5. Remove from oven and let it cool completely on a wire rack.

For Assembling the Tart:
1. Once the crust has cooled, spread Greek yogurt or custard evenly over the crust.
2. Arrange assorted fresh fruits on top of the filling in an attractive pattern.
3. In a small saucepan, heat apricot preserves or honey until melted and smooth.
4. Gently brush the glaze over the arranged fruits for a glossy finish.
5. Chill the tart in the refrigerator for at least 1 hour before serving to set.

Nutritional Information (per serving)
- Calories: 250
- Protein: 6g
- Carbohydrates: 30g
- Fiber: 5g
- Fat: 14g

Tips for Making it Low Uric Acid-Friendly
- Opt for low-fat Greek yogurt or custard to reduce saturated fat.
- Choose fresh fruits that are lower in purines, such as berries and kiwi.

9. Frozen Yogurt with Honey and Blueberries

Intro: Frozen yogurt with honey and blueberries is a light and refreshing dessert that combines the tanginess of yogurt with the sweetness of honey and antioxidant-rich blueberries.

Total Prep Time

- 5 minutes (plus freezing time)

Ingredients

- 2 cups Greek yogurt
- 1/4 cup honey
- 1 cup fresh blueberries

Instructions

1. In a bowl, mix Greek yogurt and honey until well combined.
2. Gently fold in fresh blueberries.
3. Transfer the mixture to a freezer-safe container.
4. Freeze for 2-3 hours, stirring occasionally, until firm.
5. Scoop frozen yogurt into bowls and serve immediately.

Nutritional Information (per serving)

- Calories: 200
- Protein: 15g
- Carbohydrates: 30g
- Fiber: 2g
- Fat: 0g

Tips for Making it Low Uric Acid-Friendly

- Greek yogurt is low in purines and high in protein.
- Use natural honey sparingly for sweetness.

10. Peach and Raspberry Crumble

Intro: Peach and raspberry crumble is a comforting and fruity dessert topped with a crunchy oat and almond topping, perfect for enjoying warm with a dollop of yogurt or a scoop of vanilla ice cream.

Total Prep Time

- 45 minutes

Ingredients
For the Fruit Filling:
- 4 cups sliced peaches (fresh or frozen)
- 2 cups raspberries (fresh or frozen)
- 1/4 cup honey or maple syrup
- 1 tablespoon lemon juice
- 2 tablespoons cornstarch

For the Crumble Topping:
- 1 cup rolled oats
- 1/2 cup almond flour
- 1/4 cup chopped almonds
- 1/4 cup coconut oil, melted
- 1/4 cup honey or maple syrup
- 1 teaspoon ground cinnamon

Instructions
For the Fruit Filling:
1. Preheat the oven to 350°F (175°C). Grease a baking dish.
2. In a large bowl, combine sliced peaches, raspberries, honey or maple syrup, lemon juice, and cornstarch. Toss until fruit is coated evenly.
3. Transfer the fruit mixture to the prepared baking dish, spreading it out evenly.

For the Crumble Topping:
1. In a separate bowl, mix rolled oats, almond flour, chopped almonds, melted coconut oil, honey or maple syrup, and ground cinnamon until crumbly.
2. Sprinkle the crumble mixture evenly over the fruit filling in the baking dish.
3. Bake for 30-35 minutes, until the fruit is bubbling and the crumble topping is golden brown.
4. Remove from oven and let it cool for 10 minutes before serving.
5. Serve warm, optionally with a scoop of yogurt or ice cream.

Nutritional Information (per serving)

- Calories: 300
- Protein: 6g
- Carbohydrates: 50g
- Fiber: 6g
- Fat: 10g

Tips for Making it Low Uric Acid-Friendly
- Use almond flour and oats for the crumble topping instead of traditional flour.
- Limit added sugars by reducing the amount of honey or maple syrup.

11. Avocado Chocolate Mousse

Intro: Avocado chocolate mousse is a silky and indulgent dessert made with ripe avocados and dark chocolate, offering a rich flavor and creamy texture without dairy or added sugars.

Total Prep Time
- 15 minutes (plus chilling time)

Ingredients
- 2 ripe avocados, peeled and pitted
- 1/2 cup cocoa powder (unsweetened)
- 1/4 cup honey or maple syrup
- 1 teaspoon vanilla extract
- 1/4 cup almond milk (unsweetened)

Instructions
1. In a blender or food processor, combine peeled and pitted avocados, cocoa powder, honey or maple syrup, vanilla extract, and almond milk.
2. Blend until smooth and creamy, scraping down the sides as needed.
3. Transfer mousse to serving dishes or bowls.
4. Chill in the refrigerator for at least 1 hour to set.
5. Serve chilled, optionally garnished with fresh berries or shaved chocolate.

Nutritional Information (per serving)
- Calories: 250

- Protein: 5g
- Carbohydrates: 30g
- Fiber: 10g
- Fat: 15g

Tips for Making it Low Uric Acid-Friendly

- Avocados are low in purines and provide healthy fats.
- Use unsweetened cocoa powder and limit added sweeteners.

12. Pumpkin Pie with Whole Grain Crust

Intro: Pumpkin pie with whole grain crust is a classic dessert with a wholesome twist, featuring a spiced pumpkin filling and a nutty whole grain crust that's perfect for autumn gatherings.

Total Prep Time

- 1 hour 30 minutes

Ingredients

For the Whole Grain Crust:

- 1 1/2 cups whole wheat flour
- 1/2 cup almond flour
- 1/4 cup coconut oil, melted
- 2 tablespoons honey or maple syrup
- 1/4 cup cold water

For the Pumpkin Filling:

- 1 can (15 oz) pumpkin puree
- 1/2 cup coconut milk (full-fat)
- 1/2 cup honey or maple syrup
- 2 eggs
- 1 teaspoon vanilla extract
- 1 teaspoon ground cinnamon
- 1/2 teaspoon ground nutmeg
- 1/4 teaspoon ground cloves
- 1/4 teaspoon salt

Instructions

For the Whole Grain Crust:

1. Preheat the oven to 350°F (175°C). Grease a pie dish.
2. In a bowl, mix whole wheat flour, almond flour, melted coconut oil, honey or maple syrup, and cold water until dough forms.
3. Press the dough evenly into the bottom and up the sides of the greased pie dish.
4. Bake the crust for 10-12 minutes, until lightly golden brown. Remove from oven and set aside.

For the Pumpkin Filling:

1. In a large bowl, whisk together pumpkin puree, coconut milk, honey or maple syrup, eggs, vanilla extract, ground cinnamon, ground nutmeg, ground cloves, and salt until smooth.
2. Pour pumpkin filling into the pre-baked pie crust.
3. Bake for 50-60 minutes, until the center is set.
4. Remove from oven and let the pie cool completely on a wire rack.
5. Chill in the refrigerator for at least 2 hours before serving.

Nutritional Information (per serving)

- Calories: 300
- Protein: 6g
- Carbohydrates: 45g
- Fiber: 5g
- Fat: 12g

Tips for Making it Low Uric Acid-Friendly

- Use whole wheat and almond flour for the crust to increase fiber content.
- Limit added sugars by adjusting the amount of honey or maple syrup.

13. Lemon and Blueberry Cheesecake

Intro: Lemon and blueberry cheesecake is a delightful dessert that blends the zesty flavors of lemon with the sweetness of blueberries, all atop a crunchy graham cracker crust.

Total Prep Time

- 1 hour 30 minutes (plus chilling time)

Ingredients

For the Graham Cracker Crust:

- 1 1/2 cups graham cracker crumbs
- 1/4 cup coconut oil, melted
- 2 tablespoons honey or maple syrup

For the Cheesecake Filling:

- 16 ounces cream cheese, softened
- 1 cup Greek yogurt
- 1/2 cup honey or maple syrup
- Zest and juice of 1 lemon
- 2 eggs
- 1 teaspoon vanilla extract

For the Blueberry Topping:

- 1 cup fresh blueberries
- 2 tablespoons honey or maple syrup
- 1 tablespoon water
- 1 teaspoon cornstarch

Instructions

For the Graham Cracker Crust:

1. Preheat the oven to 350°F (175°C). Grease a 9-inch springform pan.
2. In a bowl, combine graham cracker crumbs, melted coconut oil, and honey or maple syrup until well mixed.
3. Press the mixture evenly into the bottom of the prepared pan.
4. Bake the crust for 8-10 minutes, until lightly golden brown. Remove from oven and set aside to cool.

For the Cheesecake Filling:

1. In a large mixing bowl, beat softened cream cheese until smooth and creamy.
2. Add Greek yogurt, honey or maple syrup, lemon zest, lemon juice, eggs, and vanilla extract. Beat until well combined and smooth.

3. Pour the cheesecake filling over the cooled graham cracker crust in the springform pan.
4. Smooth the top with a spatula.

For the Blueberry Topping:

1. In a small saucepan, combine fresh blueberries, honey or maple syrup, water, and cornstarch.
2. Cook over medium heat, stirring occasionally, until the mixture thickens and blueberries soften, about 5-7 minutes.
3. Remove from heat and let it cool slightly.
4. Spread the blueberry topping evenly over the cheesecake filling.
5. Return the cheesecake to the oven and bake for 45-50 minutes, until the center is set but slightly jiggly.
6. Remove from oven and let the cheesecake cool completely on a wire rack.
7. Chill in the refrigerator for at least 4 hours or overnight before serving.

Nutritional Information (per serving)

- Calories: 350
- Protein: 8g
- Carbohydrates: 35g
- Fiber: 2g
- Fat: 20g

Tips for Making it Low Uric Acid-Friendly

- Use low-fat cream cheese or Greek yogurt to reduce saturated fat content.
- Opt for natural sweeteners like honey or maple syrup in moderation.

14. Strawberry and Basil Sorbet

Intro: Strawberry and basil sorbet is a refreshing and herbaceous dessert that combines the sweetness of strawberries with the aromatic essence of fresh basil, perfect for a light and cooling treat.

Total Prep Time

- 5 minutes (plus freezing time)

Ingredients

- 4 cups fresh strawberries, hulled
- 1/2 cup fresh basil leaves
- 1/4 cup honey or agave syrup
- 1 tablespoon lemon juice

Instructions

1. In a blender or food processor, combine fresh strawberries, basil leaves, honey or agave syrup, and lemon juice.
2. Blend until smooth and well combined.
3. Taste and adjust sweetness if necessary.
4. Pour the mixture into a shallow dish and freeze for 4-6 hours, stirring occasionally, until firm.
5. Scoop sorbet into bowls and serve immediately.

Nutritional Information (per serving)

- Calories: 150
- Protein: 1g
- Carbohydrates: 35g
- Fiber: 4g
- Fat: 0g

Tips for Making it Low Uric Acid-Friendly

- Strawberries are low in purines and high in vitamin C.
- Use natural sweeteners and avoid artificial additives.

15. Baked Pears with Walnuts and Honey

Intro: Baked pears with walnuts and honey are a simple yet elegant dessert that highlights the natural sweetness of pears, complemented by crunchy walnuts and a drizzle of honey.

Total Prep Time

- 30 minutes

Ingredients

- 4 ripe but firm pears, halved and cored
- 1/2 cup walnuts, chopped
- 2 tablespoons honey

- 1 teaspoon ground cinnamon

Instructions
1. Preheat the oven to 375°F (190°C). Grease a baking dish.
2. Place pear halves cut side up in the baking dish.
3. In a small bowl, mix chopped walnuts, honey, and ground cinnamon until well combined.
4. Spoon the walnut mixture evenly into the hollowed-out center of each pear half.
5. Cover the baking dish with foil and bake for 20 minutes.
6. Remove foil and bake for an additional 10 minutes, until pears are tender and topping is golden brown.
7. Remove from oven and let it cool slightly before serving.

Nutritional Information (per serving)
- Calories: 200
- Protein: 3g
- Carbohydrates: 30g
- Fiber: 5g
- Fat: 10g

Tips for Making it Low Uric Acid-Friendly
- Pears are low in purines and rich in dietary fiber.
- Use natural honey sparingly for sweetness.

These recipes offer a variety of delicious and nutritious desserts while keeping considerations for a low uric acid diet in mind.

5.6 Smoothie Recipes

1. Mango and Turmeric Smoothie
Intro: Mango and turmeric smoothie is a vibrant and refreshing blend that combines the tropical sweetness of mango with the anti-inflammatory benefits of turmeric.

Total Prep Time
- 5 minutes

Ingredients

- 1 cup frozen mango chunks
- 1/2 teaspoon ground turmeric
- 1 cup coconut water or almond milk
- 1 tablespoon honey or agave syrup (optional)

Instructions

1. In a blender, combine frozen mango chunks, ground turmeric, coconut water or almond milk, and honey or agave syrup.
2. Blend until smooth and creamy.
3. Taste and adjust sweetness if necessary.
4. Pour into glasses and serve immediately.

Nutritional Information (per serving)

- Calories: 150
- Protein: 1g
- Carbohydrates: 35g
- Fiber: 4g
- Fat: 1g

Tips for Making it Low Uric Acid-Friendly

- Mango is low in purines and adds natural sweetness.
- Use coconut water instead of almond milk to reduce purine intake.

2. Green Detox Smoothie

Intro: Green detox smoothie is a nutrient-packed drink that helps cleanse and refresh your body with the goodness of leafy greens and hydrating ingredients.

Total Prep Time

- 7 minutes

Ingredients

- 1 cup spinach
- 1/2 cup kale leaves
- 1/2 cucumber, peeled and chopped
- 1 green apple, cored and chopped

- Juice of 1 lemon
- 1 cup coconut water or plain water

Instructions

1. In a blender, combine spinach, kale leaves, cucumber, green apple, lemon juice, and coconut water or water.
2. Blend until smooth and creamy.
3. Taste and adjust flavor as needed.
4. Pour into glasses and serve immediately.

Nutritional Information (per serving)

- Calories: 120
- Protein: 3g
- Carbohydrates: 30g
- Fiber: 7g
- Fat: 1g

Tips for Making it Low Uric Acid-Friendly

- Leafy greens like spinach and kale are low in purines and high in antioxidants.
- Use coconut water for added hydration without purines found in dairy.

3. Pineapple and Kale Smoothie

Intro: Pineapple and kale smoothie is a tropical delight packed with vitamins, minerals, and enzymes that support digestion and boost immunity.

Total Prep Time

- 5 minutes

Ingredients

- 1 cup fresh pineapple chunks
- 1 cup kale leaves, chopped
- 1 banana, peeled
- 1/2 cup coconut water or almond milk

Instructions

1. In a blender, combine fresh pineapple chunks, kale leaves, banana, and coconut water or almond milk.
2. Blend until smooth and creamy.
3. Adjust consistency by adding more liquid if needed.
4. Pour into glasses and serve immediately.

Nutritional Information (per serving)

- Calories: 160
- Protein: 3g
- Carbohydrates: 40g
- Fiber: 5g
- Fat: 1g

Tips for Making it Low Uric Acid-Friendly

- Pineapple is low in purines and adds natural sweetness.
- Use coconut water instead of almond milk for a purine-free option.

4. Blueberry and Oat Smoothie

Intro: Blueberry and oat smoothie is a hearty and filling drink that combines antioxidant-rich blueberries with fiber-packed oats for a nutritious start to your day.

Total Prep Time

- 7 minutes

Ingredients

- 1 cup fresh or frozen blueberries
- 1/2 cup rolled oats
- 1 tablespoon chia seeds
- 1 cup almond milk or yogurt
- 1 tablespoon honey or maple syrup (optional)

Instructions

1. In a blender, combine blueberries, rolled oats, chia seeds, almond milk or yogurt, and honey or maple syrup.
2. Blend until smooth and creamy.
3. Adjust sweetness and thickness by adding more liquid if needed.
4. Pour into glasses and serve immediately.

Nutritional Information (per serving)
- Calories: 250
- Protein: 7g
- Carbohydrates: 45g
- Fiber: 10g
- Fat: 5g

Tips for Making it Low Uric Acid-Friendly
- Blueberries are low in purines and high in antioxidants.
- Use almond milk instead of yogurt to reduce saturated fat.

5. Strawberry and Banana Smoothie
Intro: Strawberry and banana smoothie is a classic combination that offers a creamy texture and sweet flavor, perfect for a quick and nutritious breakfast or snack.

Total Prep Time
- 5 minutes

Ingredients
- 1 cup fresh or frozen strawberries
- 1 ripe banana
- 1/2 cup Greek yogurt or coconut milk
- 1 tablespoon honey or agave syrup (optional)

Instructions
1. In a blender, combine strawberries, banana, Greek yogurt or coconut milk, and honey or agave syrup.
2. Blend until smooth and creamy.
3. Adjust sweetness and consistency by adding more liquid if needed.
4. Pour into glasses and serve immediately.

Nutritional Information (per serving)
- Calories: 200
- Protein: 6g
- Carbohydrates: 40g
- Fiber: 5g

- Fat: 2g

Tips for Making it Low Uric Acid-Friendly
- Strawberries and bananas are low in purines and high in vitamins.
- Use Greek yogurt for added protein and probiotics.

6. Avocado and Coconut Smoothie

Intro: Avocado and coconut smoothie is a creamy and nutritious blend that combines the healthy fats of avocado with the hydrating properties of coconut water for a refreshing treat.

Total Prep Time
- 5 minutes

Ingredients
- 1 ripe avocado, peeled and pitted
- 1 cup coconut water
- Juice of 1 lime
- 1 tablespoon honey or agave syrup (optional)

Instructions
1. In a blender, combine ripe avocado, coconut water, lime juice, and honey or agave syrup.
2. Blend until smooth and creamy.
3. Taste and adjust sweetness if necessary.
4. Pour into glasses and serve immediately.

Nutritional Information (per serving)
- Calories: 250
- Protein: 3g
- Carbohydrates: 25g
- Fiber: 10g
- Fat: 15g

Tips for Making it Low Uric Acid-Friendly
- Avocado is low in purines and provides healthy monounsaturated fats.
- Use coconut water for hydration without purines found in dairy.

7. Peach and Ginger Smoothie

Intro: Peach and ginger smoothie is a refreshing blend that combines the sweetness of peaches with the spicy kick of ginger, offering a burst of flavors and nutrients.

Total Prep Time

- 5 minutes

Ingredients

- 2 ripe peaches, pitted and chopped
- 1-inch piece of fresh ginger, peeled and grated
- 1/2 cup Greek yogurt or almond milk
- 1 tablespoon honey or agave syrup (optional)

Instructions

1. In a blender, combine chopped peaches, grated ginger, Greek yogurt or almond milk, and honey or agave syrup.
2. Blend until smooth and creamy.
3. Adjust sweetness and consistency by adding more liquid if needed.
4. Pour into glasses and serve immediately.

Nutritional Information (per serving)

- Calories: 180
- Protein: 5g
- Carbohydrates: 35g
- Fiber: 4g
- Fat: 3g

Tips for Making it Low Uric Acid-Friendly

- Peaches are low in purines and high in vitamins A and C.
- Use Greek yogurt for added protein or almond milk for a dairy-free option.

8. Orange and Carrot Smoothie

Intro: Orange and carrot smoothie is a vitamin-packed drink that combines the sweetness of oranges with the earthiness of carrots, offering a refreshing and nutritious boost.

Total Prep Time

- 5 minutes

Ingredients

- 2 large oranges, peeled and segmented
- 1 large carrot, peeled and chopped
- 1/2 cup coconut water or orange juice
- 1 tablespoon honey or agave syrup (optional)

Instructions

1. In a blender, combine orange segments, chopped carrot, coconut water or orange juice, and honey or agave syrup.
2. Blend until smooth and creamy.
3. Adjust sweetness and consistency by adding more liquid if needed.
4. Pour into glasses and serve immediately.

Nutritional Information (per serving)

- Calories: 150
- Protein: 3g
- Carbohydrates: 35g
- Fiber: 5g
- Fat: 1g

Tips for Making it Low Uric Acid-Friendly

- Oranges and carrots are low in purines and high in vitamin C.
- Use coconut water for hydration or orange juice for added sweetness.

9. Cucumber and Mint Smoothie

Intro: Cucumber and mint smoothie is a cooling and hydrating drink that combines crisp cucumber with refreshing mint, perfect for hot days or as a post-workout refreshment.

Total Prep Time

- 5 minutes

Ingredients

- 1 cucumber, peeled and chopped
- Handful of fresh mint leaves
- Juice of 1 lime

- 1 cup coconut water or plain water
- 1 tablespoon honey or agave syrup (optional)

Instructions

1. In a blender, combine chopped cucumber, fresh mint leaves, lime juice, add coconut water or plain water and honey or agave syrup to the blender.
2. Blend until smooth and creamy.
3. Taste and adjust sweetness if necessary.
4. Pour into glasses and garnish with a mint sprig.

Nutritional Information (per serving)

- Calories: 80
- Protein: 2g
- Carbohydrates: 20g
- Fiber: 3g
- Fat: 0g

Tips for Making it Low Uric Acid-Friendly

- Cucumber is low in purines and high in water content, aiding in hydration.
- Use coconut water instead of plain water for added electrolytes.

10. Apple Cinnamon Smoothie

Intro: Apple cinnamon smoothie is a comforting blend that combines the sweetness of apples with the warm spice of cinnamon, reminiscent of a delicious apple pie.

Total Prep Time

- 5 minutes

Ingredients

- 2 apples, cored and chopped
- 1 teaspoon ground cinnamon
- 1 cup almond milk or Greek yogurt
- 1 tablespoon honey or maple syrup (optional)
- Ice cubes (optional)

Instructions

1. In a blender, combine chopped apples, ground cinnamon, almond milk or Greek yogurt, and honey or maple syrup.
2. Add ice cubes if desired for a chilled smoothie.
3. Blend until smooth and creamy.
4. Adjust sweetness and consistency by adding more liquid if needed.
5. Pour into glasses and serve immediately.

Nutritional Information (per serving)

- Calories: 180
- Protein: 5g
- Carbohydrates: 40g
- Fiber: 7g
- Fat: 3g

Tips for Making it Low Uric Acid-Friendly

- Apples are low in purines and high in dietary fiber.
- Use almond milk instead of Greek yogurt to reduce saturated fat intake.

11. Raspberry and Chia Seed Smoothie

Intro: Raspberry and chia seed smoothie is a nutrient-dense drink that combines the tartness of raspberries with the omega-3 fatty acids and fiber from chia seeds.

Total Prep Time

- 5 minutes

Ingredients

- 1 cup fresh or frozen raspberries
- 1 tablespoon chia seeds
- 1 cup coconut water or almond milk
- Juice of 1 lemon
- 1 tablespoon honey or agave syrup (optional)

Instructions

1. In a blender, combine raspberries, chia seeds, coconut water or almond milk, lemon juice, and honey or agave syrup.
2. Blend until smooth and creamy.

3. Adjust sweetness and thickness by adding more liquid if needed.
4. Pour into glasses and serve immediately.

Nutritional Information (per serving)

- Calories: 150
- Protein: 3g
- Carbohydrates: 30g
- Fiber: 10g
- Fat: 3g

Tips for Making it Low Uric Acid-Friendly

- Raspberries are low in purines and high in antioxidants.
- Use coconut water for hydration without purines found in dairy.

12. Banana and Peanut Butter Smoothie

Intro: Banana and peanut butter smoothie is a creamy and indulgent blend that combines the sweetness of bananas with the richness of peanut butter, perfect for a quick breakfast or snack.

Total Prep Time

- 5 minutes

Ingredients

- 2 ripe bananas
- 2 tablespoons natural peanut butter
- 1 cup almond milk or Greek yogurt
- 1 tablespoon honey or maple syrup (optional)

Instructions

1. In a blender, combine ripe bananas, natural peanut butter, almond milk or Greek yogurt, and honey or maple syrup.
2. Blend until smooth and creamy.
3. Adjust sweetness and consistency by adding more liquid if needed.
4. Pour into glasses and serve immediately.

Nutritional Information (per serving)

- Calories: 300
- Protein: 8g
- Carbohydrates: 45g

- Fiber: 6g
- Fat: 10g

Tips for Making it Low Uric Acid-Friendly

- Bananas are low in purines and provide natural sweetness.
- Use almond milk instead of Greek yogurt for a dairy-free option.

13. Coconut and Lime Smoothie

Intro: Coconut and lime smoothie is a tropical delight that combines the creamy texture of coconut with the tangy freshness of lime, creating a refreshing and hydrating drink.

Total Prep Time

- 5 minutes

Ingredients

- 1 cup coconut milk
- Juice and zest of 2 limes
- 1 tablespoon honey or agave syrup (optional)
- Ice cubes (optional)

Instructions

1. In a blender, combine coconut milk, lime juice and zest, and honey or agave syrup.
2. Add ice cubes if desired for a chilled smoothie.
3. Blend until smooth and creamy.
4. Taste and adjust sweetness if necessary.
5. Pour into glasses and serve immediately.

Nutritional Information (per serving)

- Calories: 200
- Protein: 2g
- Carbohydrates: 20g
- Fiber: 1g
- Fat: 15g

Tips for Making it Low Uric Acid-Friendly

- Coconut milk is low in purines and adds a creamy texture without dairy.

- Use lime juice for a burst of citrus flavor without additional sugars.

14. Watermelon and Mint Smoothie

Intro: Watermelon and mint smoothie is a refreshing and hydrating drink that combines juicy watermelon with cooling mint, perfect for hot summer days or post-exercise recovery.

Total Prep Time

- 5 minutes

Ingredients

- 2 cups seedless watermelon, cubed
- Handful of fresh mint leaves
- Juice of 1 lime
- 1/2 cup coconut water or plain water
- 1 tablespoon honey or agave syrup (optional)

Instructions

1. In a blender, combine cubed watermelon, fresh mint leaves, lime juice, coconut water or plain water, and honey or agave syrup.
2. Blend until smooth and creamy.
3. Adjust sweetness and consistency by adding more liquid if needed.
4. Pour into glasses and serve immediately.

Nutritional Information (per serving)

- Calories: 100
- Protein: 1g
- Carbohydrates: 25g
- Fiber: 1g
- Fat: 0g

Tips for Making it Low Uric Acid-Friendly

- Watermelon is low in purines and high in water content, aiding in hydration.
- Use coconut water for added electrolytes and hydration.

15. Ginger and Pear Smoothie

Intro: Ginger and pear smoothie is a refreshing and flavorful blend that combines the sweetness of ripe pears with the spicy kick of fresh ginger, offering a unique and invigorating taste experience.

Total Prep Time

- 5 minutes

Ingredients

- 2 ripe pears, cored and chopped
- 1-inch piece of fresh ginger, peeled and grated
- 1 cup almond milk or coconut water
- Juice of 1 lemon
- 1 tablespoon honey or agave syrup (optional)

Instructions

1. In a blender, combine chopped pears, grated ginger, almond milk or coconut water, lemon juice, and honey or agave syrup.
2. Blend until smooth and creamy.
3. Taste and adjust sweetness if necessary.
4. Pour into glasses and serve immediately.

Nutritional Information (per serving)

- Calories: 180
- Protein: 2g
- Carbohydrates: 40g
- Fiber: 8g
- Fat: 2g

Tips for Making it Low Uric Acid-Friendly

- Pears are low in purines and provide natural sweetness.
- Use almond milk instead of coconut water for a creamy texture with less sugar.

These smoothie recipes offer a variety of flavors and healthy nutritional benefits while being mindful of a low uric acid diet.

CHAPTER 6:

HEALTHY 6-WEEK MEAL PLAN FOR A LOW URIC ACID DIET

6.1 Week 1

Monday
- **Breakfast**: Spinach and Mushroom Egg White Omelette
- **Lunch**: Grilled Chicken Salad with Avocado and Citrus Dressing
- **Dinner**: Baked Cod with Lemon and Dill
- **Snack**: Apple Slices with Almond Butter
- **Dessert**: Chia Seed Pudding with Coconut Milk
- **Smoothie**: Mango and Turmeric Smoothie

Tuesday
- **Breakfast**: Whole Grain Toast with Avocado and Tomato
- **Lunch**: Quinoa and Black Bean Salad with Lime Vinaigrette
- **Dinner**: Quinoa-Stuffed Bell Peppers
- **Snack**: Hummus with Carrot and Cucumber Sticks
- **Dessert**: Mixed Berry Parfait with Greek Yogurt
- **Smoothie**: Green Detox Smoothie

Wednesday
- **Breakfast**: Greek Yogurt with Honey and Walnuts
- **Lunch**: Roasted Vegetable Wrap with Hummus
- **Dinner**: Grilled Tofu with Sesame and Ginger
- **Snack**: Mixed Nuts and Dried Fruit Trail Mix
- **Dessert**: Baked Apples with Cinnamon and Raisins
- **Smoothie**: Pineapple and Kale Smoothie

Thursday
- **Breakfast**: Banana and Blueberry Smoothie Bowl
- **Lunch**: Spinach and Strawberry Salad with Poppy Seed Dressing

- **Dinner**: Baked Chicken with Rosemary and Sweet Potatoes
- **Snack**: Baked Kale Chips
- **Dessert**: Mango Sorbet
- **Smoothie**: Blueberry and Oat Smoothie

Friday

- **Breakfast**: Quinoa Breakfast Porridge with Almond Milk
- **Lunch**: Lentil and Vegetable Soup
- **Dinner**: Vegetarian Chili with Kidney Beans
- **Snack**: Greek Yogurt with Honey and Blueberries
- **Dessert**: Dark Chocolate and Walnut Bark
- **Smoothie**: Strawberry and Banana Smoothie

Saturday

- **Breakfast**: Apple Cinnamon Overnight Oats
- **Lunch**: Greek Salad with Feta and Olives
- **Dinner**: Miso Soup with Tofu and Seaweed
- **Snack**: Rice Cakes with Avocado and Tomato
- **Dessert**: Banana and Almond Butter Ice Cream
- **Smoothie**: Avocado and Coconut Smoothie

Sunday

- **Breakfast**: Chia Seed Pudding with Mixed Fruits
- **Lunch**: Grilled Salmon with Asparagus and Lemon
- **Dinner**: Stuffed Eggplant with Couscous and Herbs
- **Snack**: Roasted Chickpeas with Spices
- **Dessert**: Coconut Rice Pudding
- **Smoothie**: Peach and Ginger Smoothie

6.2 Week 2

Monday

- **Breakfast**: Scrambled Tofu with Vegetables
- **Lunch**: Chickpea and Tomato Salad with Basil
- **Dinner**: Grilled Shrimp with Garlic and Lemon
- **Snack**: Sliced Bell Peppers with Hummus
- **Dessert**: Fresh Fruit Tart with Almond Crust

- **Smoothie**: Orange and Carrot Smoothie

Tuesday

- **Breakfast**: Whole Wheat Pancakes with Maple Syrup
- **Lunch**: Whole Grain Pasta Salad with Fresh Vegetables
- **Dinner**: Lentil Stew with Carrots and Celery
- **Snack**: Celery Sticks with Peanut Butter
- **Dessert**: Frozen Yogurt with Honey and Blueberries
- **Smoothie**: Cucumber and Mint Smoothie

Wednesday

- **Breakfast**: Baked Sweet Potato and Black Bean Hash
- **Lunch**: Stuffed Bell Peppers with Quinoa and Vegetables
- **Dinner**: Roasted Cauliflower Steaks with Tahini Sauce
- **Snack**: Fresh Fruit Salad with Mint
- **Dessert**: Peach and Raspberry Crumble
- **Smoothie**: Apple Cinnamon Smoothie

Thursday

- **Breakfast**: Green Smoothie with Spinach, Kale, and Pineapple
- **Lunch**: Vegetable Stir-Fry with Brown Rice
- **Dinner**: Zucchini Noodles with Pesto Sauce
- **Snack**: Whole Grain Crackers with Cheese
- **Dessert**: Avocado Chocolate Mousse
- **Smoothie**: Raspberry and Chia Seed Smoothie

Friday

- **Breakfast**: Buckwheat Pancakes with Fresh Berries
- **Lunch**: Cucumber and Avocado Sushi Rolls
- **Dinner**: Turkey Meatballs with Spaghetti Squash
- **Snack**: Edamame with Sea Salt
- **Dessert**: Pumpkin Pie with Whole Grain Crust
- **Smoothie**: Banana and Peanut Butter Smoothie

Saturday

- **Breakfast**: Cottage Cheese with Fresh Peaches
- **Lunch**: Butternut Squash Soup with Whole Grain Bread
- **Dinner**: Sautéed Kale and White Beans
- **Snack**: Homemade Popcorn with Nutritional Yeast

- **Dessert**: Lemon and Blueberry Cheesecake
- **Smoothie**: Coconut and Lime Smoothie

Sunday

- **Breakfast**: Almond Butter and Banana on Whole Grain Toast
- **Lunch**: Mixed Greens with Balsamic Vinaigrette and Walnuts
- **Dinner**: Broiled Tilapia with Steamed Broccoli
- **Snack**: Cottage Cheese with Pineapple
- **Dessert**: Strawberry and Basil Sorbet
- **Smoothie**: Watermelon and Mint Smoothie

6.3 Week 3

Monday

- **Breakfast**: Herbed Greek Yogurt with Cucumber and Tomato Salad
- **Lunch**: Eggplant and Zucchini Ratatouille
- **Dinner**: Butternut Squash Risotto
- **Snack**: Baked Sweet Potato Fries
- **Dessert**: Baked Pears with Walnuts and Honey
- **Smoothie**: Ginger and Pear Smoothie

Tuesday

- **Breakfast**: Poached Eggs on Whole Grain English Muffin
- **Lunch**: Turkey and Avocado Lettuce Wraps
- **Dinner**: Chickpea and Spinach Curry
- **Snack**: Apple Slices with Almond Butter
- **Dessert**: Chia Seed Pudding with Coconut Milk
- **Smoothie**: Mango and Turmeric Smoothie

Wednesday

- **Breakfast**: Homemade Granola with Dried Fruits
- **Lunch**: Cauliflower Rice with Grilled Chicken and Veggies
- **Dinner**: Grilled Vegetable Skewers with Quinoa
- **Snack**: Hummus with Carrot and Cucumber Sticks
- **Dessert**: Mixed Berry Parfait with Greek Yogurt
- **Smoothie**: Green Detox Smoothie

Thursday
- **Breakfast**: Pumpkin Spice Oatmeal
- **Lunch**: Bean and Corn Salad with Cilantro Dressing
- **Dinner**: Roasted Brussels Sprouts and Chicken Thighs
- **Snack**: Mixed Nuts and Dried Fruit Trail Mix
- **Dessert**: Baked Apples with Cinnamon and Raisins
- **Smoothie**: Pineapple and Kale Smoothie

Friday
- **Breakfast**: Spinach and Feta Stuffed Whole Grain Crepes
- **Lunch**: Tomato Basil Soup with Whole Grain Crackers
- **Dinner**: Herbed Lentil and Brown Rice Pilaf
- **Snack**: Baked Kale Chips
- **Dessert**: Mango Sorbet
- **Smoothie**: Blueberry and Oat Smoothie

Saturday
- **Breakfast**: Oatmeal with Fresh Berries and Almonds
- **Lunch**: Roasted Beet and Goat Cheese Salad
- **Dinner**: Sweet and Sour Tempeh with Pineapple
- **Snack**: Greek Yogurt with Honey and Blueberries
- **Dessert**: Dark Chocolate and Walnut Bark
- **Smoothie**: Strawberry and Banana Smoothie

Sunday
- **Breakfast**: Scrambled Tofu with Vegetables
- **Lunch**: Grilled Chicken Salad with Avocado and Citrus Dressing
- **Dinner**: Baked Cod with Lemon and Dill
- **Snack**: Rice Cakes with Avocado and Tomato
- **Dessert**: Banana and Almond Butter Ice Cream
- **Smoothie**: Avocado and Coconut Smoothie

6.4 Week 4

Monday
- **Breakfast**: Whole Grain Toast with Avocado and Tomato
- **Lunch**: Quinoa and Black Bean Salad with Lime Vinaigrette

- **Dinner**: Quinoa-Stuffed Bell Peppers
- **Snack**: Roasted Chickpeas with Spices
- **Dessert**: Coconut Rice Pudding
- **Smoothie**: Peach and Ginger Smoothie

Tuesday

- **Breakfast**: Greek Yogurt with Honey and Walnuts
- **Lunch**: Roasted Vegetable Wrap with Hummus
- **Dinner**: Grilled Tofu with Sesame and Ginger
- **Snack**: Sliced Bell Peppers with Hummus
- **Dessert**: Fresh Fruit Tart with Almond Crust
- **Smoothie**: Orange and Carrot Smoothie

Wednesday

- **Breakfast**: Banana and Blueberry Smoothie Bowl
- **Lunch**: Spinach and Strawberry Salad with Poppy Seed Dressing
- **Dinner**: Baked Chicken with Rosemary and Sweet Potatoes
- **Snack**: Celery Sticks with Peanut Butter
- **Dessert**: Frozen Yogurt with Honey and Blueberries
- **Smoothie**: Cucumber and Mint Smoothie

Thursday

- **Breakfast**: Quinoa Breakfast Porridge with Almond Milk
- **Lunch**: Lentil and Vegetable Soup
- **Dinner**: Vegetarian Chili with Kidney Beans
- **Snack**: Fresh Fruit Salad with Mint
- **Dessert**: Peach and Raspberry Crumble
- **Smoothie**: Apple Cinnamon Smoothie

Friday

- **Breakfast**: Apple Cinnamon Overnight Oats
- **Lunch**: Greek Salad with Feta and Olives
- **Dinner**: Miso Soup with Tofu and Seaweed
- **Snack**: Whole Grain Crackers with Cheese
- **Dessert**: Avocado Chocolate Mousse
- **Smoothie**: Raspberry and Chia Seed Smoothie

Saturday

- **Breakfast**: Chia Seed Pudding with Mixed Fruits

- **Lunch**: Grilled Salmon with Asparagus and Lemon
- **Dinner**: Stuffed Eggplant with Couscous and Herbs
- **Snack**: Edamame with Sea Salt
- **Dessert**: Pumpkin Pie with Whole Grain Crust
- **Smoothie**: Banana and Peanut Butter Smoothie

Sunday
- **Breakfast**: Scrambled Tofu with Vegetables
- **Lunch**: Chickpea and Tomato Salad with Basil
- **Dinner**: Lentil Stew with Carrots and Celery
- **Snack**: Cottage Cheese with Pineapple
- **Dessert**: Lemon and Blueberry Cheesecake
- **Smoothie**: Coconut and Lime Smoothie

6.5 Week 5

Monday
- **Breakfast**: Whole Wheat Pancakes with Maple Syrup
- **Lunch**: Whole Grain Pasta Salad with Fresh Vegetables
- **Dinner**: Roasted Cauliflower Steaks with Tahini Sauce
- **Snack**: Homemade Popcorn with Nutritional Yeast
- **Dessert**: Strawberry and Basil Sorbet
- **Smoothie**: Watermelon and Mint Smoothie

Tuesday
- **Breakfast**: Baked Sweet Potato and Black Bean Hash
- **Lunch**: Stuffed Bell Peppers with Quinoa and Vegetables
- **Dinner**: Zucchini Noodles with Pesto Sauce
- **Snack**: Baked Sweet Potato Fries
- **Dessert**: Baked Pears with Walnuts and Honey
- **Smoothie**: Ginger and Pear Smoothie

Wednesday
- **Breakfast**: Green Smoothie with Spinach, Kale, and Pineapple
- **Lunch**: Vegetable Stir-Fry with Brown Rice
- **Dinner**: Turkey Meatballs with Spaghetti Squash
- **Snack**: Apple Slices with Almond Butter

- **Dessert**: Chia Seed Pudding with Coconut Milk
- **Smoothie**: Mango and Turmeric Smoothie

Thursday
- **Breakfast**: Buckwheat Pancakes with Fresh Berries
- **Lunch**: Cucumber and Avocado Sushi Rolls
- **Dinner**: Sautéed Kale and White Beans
- **Snack**: Hummus with Carrot and Cucumber Sticks
- **Dessert**: Mixed Berry Parfait with Greek Yogurt
- **Smoothie**: Green Detox Smoothie

Friday
- **Breakfast**: Cottage Cheese with Fresh Peaches
- **Lunch**: Butternut Squash Soup with Whole Grain Bread
- **Dinner**: Broiled Tilapia with Steamed Broccoli
- **Snack**: Mixed Nuts and Dried Fruit Trail Mix
- **Dessert**: Baked Apples with Cinnamon and Raisins
- **Smoothie**: Pineapple and Kale Smoothie

Saturday
- **Breakfast**: Almond Butter and Banana on Whole Grain Toast
- **Lunch**: Mixed Greens with Balsamic Vinaigrette and Walnuts
- **Dinner**: Butternut Squash Risotto
- **Snack**: Baked Kale Chips
- **Dessert**: Mango Sorbet
- **Smoothie**: Blueberry and Oat Smoothie

Sunday
- **Breakfast**: Herbed Greek Yogurt with Cucumber and Tomato Salad
- **Lunch**: Eggplant and Zucchini Ratatouille
- **Dinner**: Sweet and Sour Tempeh with Pineapple
- **Snack**: Greek Yogurt with Honey and Blueberries
- **Dessert**: Dark Chocolate and Walnut Bark
- **Smoothie**: Strawberry and Banana Smoothie

6.6 Week 6

Monday

- **Breakfast**: Poached Eggs on Whole Grain English Muffin
- **Lunch**: Turkey and Avocado Lettuce Wraps
- **Dinner**: Grilled Tofu with Sesame and Ginger
- **Snack**: Rice Cakes with Avocado and Tomato
- **Dessert**: Coconut Rice Pudding
- **Smoothie**: Peach and Ginger Smoothie

Tuesday

- **Breakfast**: Homemade Granola with Dried Fruits
- **Lunch**: Cauliflower Rice with Grilled Chicken and Veggies
- **Dinner**: Baked Chicken with Rosemary and Sweet Potatoes
- **Snack**: Roasted Chickpeas with Spices
- **Dessert**: Fresh Fruit Tart with Almond Crust
- **Smoothie**: Orange and Carrot Smoothie

Wednesday

- **Breakfast**: Pumpkin Spice Oatmeal
- **Lunch**: Bean and Corn Salad with Cilantro Dressing
- **Dinner**: Grilled Shrimp with Garlic and Lemon
- **Snack**: Sliced Bell Peppers with Hummus
- **Dessert**: Banana and Almond Butter Ice Cream
- **Smoothie**: Avocado and Coconut Smoothie

Thursday

- **Breakfast**: Spinach and Feta Stuffed Whole Grain Crepes
- **Lunch**: Tomato Basil Soup with Whole Grain Crackers
- **Dinner**: Stuffed Eggplant with Couscous and Herbs
- **Snack**: Celery Sticks with Peanut Butter
- **Dessert**: Peach and Raspberry Crumble
- **Smoothie**: Cucumber and Mint Smoothie

Friday

- **Breakfast**: Oatmeal with Fresh Berries and Almonds
- **Lunch**: Greek Salad with Feta and Olives
- **Dinner**: Lentil Stew with Carrots and Celery
- **Snack**: Edamame with Sea Salt
- **Dessert**: Avocado Chocolate Mousse

- **Smoothie**: Watermelon and Mint Smoothie

Saturday
- **Breakfast**: Spinach and Mushroom Egg White Omelette
- **Lunch**: Grilled Chicken Salad with Avocado and Citrus Dressing
- **Dinner**: Roasted Brussels Sprouts and Chicken Thighs
- **Snack**: Whole Grain Crackers with Cheese
- **Dessert**: Chia Seed Pudding with Coconut Milk
- **Smoothie**: Ginger and Pear Smoothie

Sunday
- **Breakfast**: Whole Grain Toast with Avocado and Tomato
- **Lunch**: Roasted Vegetable Wrap with Hummus
- **Dinner**: Herbed Lentil and Brown Rice Pilaf
- **Snack**: Cottage Cheese with Pineapple
- **Dessert**: Lemon and Blueberry Cheesecake
- **Smoothie**: Pineapple and Kale Smoothie

This 6-week meal plan provides a comprehensive guide to maintaining a low uric acid diet, offering a variety of meals that are both nutritious and delicious. Each day is balanced with breakfast, lunch, dinner, snacks, desserts, and smoothies, ensuring that you get all the essential nutrients while keeping your meals enjoyable and interesting.

Enjoy your meals and stay healthy!

CONCLUSION

Thank you for embarking on this culinary journey with us through the "Low Uric Acid Diet Cookbook." This book was created with the aim of transforming the way you think about food and health, making it easier and more enjoyable to manage your uric acid levels.

Navigating dietary changes can be challenging, especially when it involves managing a condition like high uric acid levels. However, with the right resources and a bit of creativity, it's possible to maintain a diet that not only supports your health but also excites your palate. This cookbook is designed to be that resource, offering you a collection of recipes that are both healthful and flavorful, ensuring that you never feel deprived while on your journey to better health.

Each recipe in this book has been thoughtfully developed to balance nutrients and taste, proving that a low uric acid diet can be varied and delicious. From hearty breakfasts that kickstart your day with energy to satisfying lunches, delectable dinners, and indulgent yet healthy desserts, this cookbook offers a full spectrum of meal options. Whether you're a seasoned cook or new to the kitchen, these recipes are accessible, easy to follow, and enjoyable to prepare.

Moreover, the "Low Uric Acid Diet Cookbook" is more than just a collection of recipes. It's a guide to adopting a lifestyle that supports your health goals. With practical tips, meal plans, and insights into managing your diet in various scenarios—be it dining out, traveling, or handling setbacks—you are well-equipped to make informed decisions and stay on track.

The benefits of following a low uric acid diet extend far beyond managing uric acid levels. You'll likely experience improved overall health, increased energy levels, and a greater sense of well-being. This journey is about embracing a lifestyle that nourishes your body and enhances your quality of life, one meal at a time.

We hope that this cookbook inspires you to explore new flavors, try new ingredients, and take pride in preparing meals that are both delicious and healthful. Remember, the key to success lies in consistency and making informed choices that align with your health goals. The recipes and tips provided in this book are designed to make this process as seamless and enjoyable as possible.

As you incorporate these recipes into your daily routine, we encourage you to listen to your body and make adjustments as needed. Everyone's journey to health is unique, and finding what works best for you is essential. This cookbook is your companion on this journey, offering support, inspiration, and delicious meals that make the path to a low uric acid lifestyle a delightful one.

Here's to a future filled with vibrant health, delicious food, and the satisfaction of knowing you're taking proactive steps to support your well-being. Enjoy the recipes, savor the flavors, and relish the journey towards a healthier, happier you. Thank you for choosing the "Low Uric Acid Diet Cookbook" as your guide to a better, more nourishing way of eating.

Patricia D. Miller